HIV AND DRUG FREE
Cancer And The
Immune System
Including Natural Therapy Recommendations

By: Eileen Renders N. D

ISBN: 0-9711551-6-X
By Eileen Renders N. D.
Renders Wellness/Publishing
Copyright 2004

(Provided by Quality Books, Inc.) Publisher's Cataloging-in-Publication

Renders, Eileen, 1939-
    HIV and drug free: cancer and the immune system/ Eileen Renders.
    p. cm.
    Includes bibliographical references and index.

    1. HIV infections — Nutritional aspects. 2. HIV-positive persons--Nutrition 3. AIDS (Disease) — Nutritional aspects. 4. AIDS (Disease)---Treatment. 5. Naturopathy.
    1. Title
RC606.6R46 2004   616.97'920654
                    QB133-1710

CONTENTS

One	Alternative Medicine Opportunity	01
Two	N.I.H. ~ National Institutes Health Provides Legitimacy To Alternative Medicine	05
Three	Renders Wellness is Sub-contracted By ACMC'S HIV Consortium	07
Four	Renders Wellness Creates And Implements HIV/AIDS Protocol	10
Five	Immediate Problematic Findings	15
Six	Initial Intake Interviews	22
Seven	Case Histories	27
Eight	General Recommendations	44
Nine	Specific Recommendations	51
Ten	Antagonists, Devitalized foods, Including Suspected Carcinogens	55
Eleven	Healthier Food Replacements	63
Twelve	Drugs s used in the Treatment Of HIV	66
Thirteen	Tracking Bernie's Progress	79
Fourteen	Cancer	99
Fifteen	The Immune System	110
Sixteen	Recipes	123

INTRODUCTION

In 1995 and immediately following the degree entitling me the designation of Doctor of Naturopathy (N.D.), Renders Wellness was founded. While most still could not pronounce Natur op athy, this was to become my new profession and chosen field of expertise. Sometime back in 1991 I became disillusioned with traditional Western medicine and began to nourish a fundamental belief that nutrition and concentrated nutrients, when supplemented in proper potency for specific disorders was the best over-looked non-toxic therapy available for most of us. They are also non-addictive and essential to our health.

This approach to wellness I had found was an approach that was also compatible with my own inner beliefs and philosophies. Admittedly however, while I have to confess to having had my own initial difficulty with pronouncing *Naturopathy,* instinctively what was gradually being revealed to me about this form of natural healing, felt comfortable to me.

While Naturopathy includes courses in Homeopathy, Reflexology, Iridology, Acupressure, Herbology as well as Nutrition, it is necessary that each individual select a "specialty" that he/she is most attracted to, before spending the hours of study and research that will be required in order to better hone one's skills. What I believed and continue to believe today is that our medical physician's are the greatest diagnosticians in the world and have at their disposal the highest technological tools enabling them to

I

adequately fulfill their responsibilities. Furthermore, as far as surgeons are concerned, it is my opinion that many a life would have been cut short were it not for their invasive intervention.

As far as medical specialists are concerned, I believe that diagnosis, treatment and monitoring of many disorders, such as diabetes or heart disease, is well within their expertise. This is especially true for the elderly, obese and or those who have followed sedentary lifestyles.

These individuals are obviously not the best candidates for seeking to make dramatic health transitions through alternative approaches. However for those who are healthy enough and willing to make gradual transitions in their life style and eating habits, they may be in for a pleasant surprise. Motivation and choice for one's directional path are well founded when compatible with one's inner beliefs. These are essential key elements to success in one's quest to success. Success is often said to be "Doing what makes one happy", or what is compatible with what one believes in. There is no greater satisfaction in life than helping others, and that comes to us through sharing of knowledge.

Furthermore, while some medications may be warranted for serious disorders, (such as antibiotics for a serious or unexplained infection) they may not always be the best approach for everyone, especially when it comes to managing a common disorder for which there is very often no cure. Yet many commonly prescribed drugs now being prescribed liberally for treating common disorders are not always well tolerated by every patient.

This very often causes the patient to experience a whole new set of side effects and symptoms as a result of these potent medications. Ironically, these new symptoms are often addressed by prescribing yet another medication. While many of these drugs may be addictive, others can often contribute to liver toxicity. Toxicities that accumulate within the liver will weaken the immune system and can contribute to a whole new disorder. An example of this is documented by the number of patients prescribed steroids for inflammatory conditions such as arthritis. When steroids are taken for an extended period of time, they can often cause ulcers that eventually lead to internal bleeding! And steroids have been shown to result in hemorrhaging which can be life threatening!

In fact, patients often build up a "tolerance' to a particular drug when it is taken over an extended period of time. What this means is that the drug soon loses its ability to affect the same benefit as it evoked earlier on in initial stages of treatment. In my own practice this is often referred to as the *snowball effect*. In other words, as tolerance to the drug increases, resistance often leads to a need for a higher potency to be prescribed, or a combination of drugs to treat the disorder.

Again, annoying or persistent symptoms from a medication that leads to yet another prescribed medication is counter-productive! Often described as a viscous, repetitive off-again, on-again cycle! At best, in the case of common disorders, prescribed drugs temporarily alleviate the symptoms without addressing the underlying cause. Often the correction of a severe nutritional deficiency will provide much benefit.

Another consideration is the Liver itself. The Liver is the body's main filtering organ and is responsible for filtering out all toxic substances (but for several prescribed drugs that are passed through the kidneys). While the Liver is forgiving to some degree, an accumulative buildup of toxins can lead to a weakened immune system. Examples of how this happens might be best understood when we see how many cancer patients being treated with aggressive chemo drugs often die not from the cancers they were fighting, but from Liver failure due to a buildup of toxicity! The Liver simply blows up, becomes inflamed and swollen and ceases to function.

Another similarity of lesser severity might be noted whenever a patient is prescribed antibiotics frequently. Antibiotics (much like Chemo drugs) do not discriminate between good bacteria and bad bacteria, therefore killing all bacterial that it comes in contact with. When this occurs, some individuals will find themselves reliving the experience for which they initially sought treatment. A rebound occurrence, or bout after bout of bacterial infection that is often treated in exactly the same manner. Yet common sense tells us that these recurrences tell us that the treatment is not working.

Candida is an example of the kind of bacterial infection of which I speak. However, in subtle ways, antibiotic therapy can be effective when the patient is recommended a high potency pro-biotic upon completion of their antibiotics. In this way, the patient is able to replenish the much-needed intestinal bacteria, or intestinal flora that protects the gut by fighting off the "bad bacteria." A good source of this is readily found at the local Health Food Store and will include L.acidophilus, Lactobacillus casei and Bifidobacterium longum.

In the case of Candida or the single cell fungus known as *Candida albicans* one needs to temporarily avoid refined white sugar, as well as most other forms of sugar. Because sugar tastes sweet to the palate, it is easy to overlook the fact that sugar is an acid. This fungus (as well as many others) thrive best in an acidic internal environment.

Another thought is to understand that very often-prescribed medications are utilized best when employed temporarily to address symptoms associated with various disorders. Because most medications offer few cures, they are not always the best therapy in management of common disorders.

Some investigational work is necessary in order to discover whether a particular disorder is genetic, environmental, or a latent problem due to significant deficiencies of essential nutrients and/or worsened due to poor nutrition, or unhealthy life style practices. Cigarette smoking, over-eating, including a sedentary life style definitely can contribute to the vulnerability of our susceptibility to a particular disease such as: Cancer, heart disease, diabetes or upper respiratory problems.

Knowledge is empowerment. We are empowered whenever we are able to discern when medical intervention is necessary, or when we might be in a good position to manage and/or reverse a specific disorder such as those often said to be "borderline."

High blood pressure is a serious disorder that requires medication in order to prevent a stroke, heart attack or death. However, a "borderline" patient is one who has slightly elevated readings, yet may be young and healthy enough to institute healthier nutritional habits, as well as a regular routine of exercise. More often than not, this will bring "borderline" hypertension back within the normal range. Type two diabetes has also been reversed or managed without drugs when the individual (who has his or her physician's approval) begins an exercise program and institutes a few subtle changes in the diet.

It is a wise individual who will get a second opinion, evaluate and review one's options and become involved in his/her health.

Professionally speaking, it is my contention that in acute or traumatic crisis only medical intervention will do. However in exploring our options in terms of management of many diagnosed common disorders, perhaps drugs may not always the best direction for each of us. Keep an open mind and explore your options, align your decision making process so that it is compatible with your inner beliefs and go forward.

Why is it that drugs created to aid, or affect a cure often cause adverse, if not toxic side effects? Perhaps this is where the Doctor of Naturopathy greatly differs with the traditional Allopath. We differ inasmuch as our philosophies and beliefs differ. For example, during a Lecture or Class, the naturopath will often point to the fact that we as humans are organic. To take that a step further let me continue by saying that every vitamin, mineral or nutrient found in the earth's rich soil and in her deepest oceans is also organic. This is exactly what makes those compounds more compatible with the human (organic) body.

Synthetic supplements and/or prescribed drugs on the other hand, are inorganic. Inorganic, or synthetic is not compatible with the human body, and is often difficult to digest and/or metabolize. All of which can lead to side effects and/or symptoms confirming an incompatibility!

Perhaps the Clergy best confirms this at the time of death of a loved one. As we stand beside the gravesite we hear the clergy utter those familiar words: "Dust thou art, and dust thou shalt return!"

However, there will always be two sides to a story and we who believe in taking part in our health management may hear someone say, "What is the point? We are all going to die anyway!" To that I would respond: "Yes, but why rush it?" Some who oppose Natural medicine might also say: "What about the athlete who didn't smoke, ate right, exercised all his life and then died suddenly at 38 years of age of a heart attack?"

Who is to say that this individual might not have spent several years as an invalid, or gone through surgery after surgery and lived out his last five years depressed with the impending doom of an early death hanging over his head had he not lived a clean life?

Friends, there are many hypothetical theories with regard to how one ought to live his or her life. Perhaps this is why one must live his/her life true to one's convictions (or inner belief's). Living a life style that is not compatible with one's inner beliefs can only foster inner conflict. And that inner conflict can lead to psychological as well as physiological stress. For sure, most of us realize by now how stress plays a big part (whether it be excessive or ongoing) in weakening the immune system. This is due to the fact that stress compromises digestion, absorption and metabolism of our essential nutrients. This wrecks havoc because in times of stress, our body actually requires more of certain nutrients, especially the B+ Complex vitamin.

Yet all of our nutrients (in times of stress) are being utilized to combat stress! Consequently, our body is less able to fight off potential problems, making us less resistant to disease. Common sense tells us that a weakened immune system lays us open and vulnerable to more serious types of disease.

Disease, now there is a word for us to ponder. Disease is that state of being when one is in dis-harmony with God and nature (or self). As a N.D. I chose two specialties, Nutritional therapy and Herbal Medicine. It seemed to me that Nutrition was the very foundation upon which man is created and nourished. Hundreds of years ago it was discovered how disease was often associated with the onset of nutritional deficiencies. One example is the Sailors who spent months at sea. Aboard Ship without proper nourishment, especially Vitamin-C, many came down with Rickets'. This disease is diagnosed by symptoms such as: Bleeding gums and weakened bones among other obvious symptoms. As soon as Vitamin C was added to their diets however, the problem slowly began to reverse itself.

A loss of Calcium, (this is not always an age related problem) perhaps due to inadequate intake, poor utilization of the mineral, or high levels of antagonistic minerals (such as either phosphorous or magnesium) could be the culprit. Maybe a menopausal woman with a detected Calcium deficiency is unknowingly compounding the problem because of her love of spinach. It has been discovered that eating a food (much like spinach) that contains a good deal of oxalic acid on a regular basis can interfere with Calcium absorption because oxalic acid and Calcium are antagonistic to one another!

Children with ADD and ADHD are often prescribed a drug (Ritalin), which can have very deleterious side effects for many children, especially when taken for extended periods of time. Side effects include: Stunted growth, insomnia, heart palpitations and other symptoms. Yet many of these same children have nutritional problems that lead to the very symptoms mentioned for confirming the diagnosis of ADD and ADHD. Yet many experts are of the opinion that often these children express hyperactive behavior as a result of improper nutrition. For example: These children often favor high sodium snack foods such as: Potato chips, pretzels, pop corn, Luncheon meats, peanuts or canned soups and highly processed macaroni and cheese.

Yet it is a known fact that Sodium chloride (Table Salt) contains a fair amount of Iodine. Excess Iodine

intake can over-stimulate the Thyroid glands, thus contributing to the hyper kinetic child. Because this is not a book about Common Disorders and the Nutritional Antagonists that can often be involved in the disease process and examples are provided only to make a point, no further elaboration is required. For more specific information from author sees Resources section in back of book (Common Disorders ~ Natural Remedies and The Holistic Cookbook). Herbal Medicine (Alternative medicine) is my second chosen Specialty because herbs are for the most part (about 98% of herbs), non-toxic. It is not meant to infer that herbs and concentrated nutrients are an over night cure or a cure at all. However, more often than not, much benefit can be derived through specific recommendations when they are made under the supervision of a skilled and credentialed practitioner. In this way, contraindications will be considered as well as duration and potency of each recommendation. Unlike a prescribed synthetic (inorganic) medication, herbs and other supplements are slower acting and require time to build up in the body's various systems, and that is the reason benefits are not always fully appreciated. It usually takes about 6 weeks before the patient can feel maximum benefit.

These recommendations are most appreciated whenever a patient has been shown to be intolerant to the usual traditional treatment. Again for some, prescription steroids may be another example of inappropriate use of a drug.

Often prescribed for treatment of allergies, yet is often seen to cause severe reactions in young children. The first sign is often a skin rash. Because steroids can have serious side effects associated with long-term use, temporary treatment might be considered, as they are not a resolution to an ongoing problem! This is one of the typical conditions that often send parents scurrying to find an alternative treatment.

Herbalists and the use of herbs go back medicinally as far as the beginning of time! They are mentioned over and over again in the Bible, regardless of which Bible you read. Hyssop, Myrrh, Olive leaf, Frankincense and other herbs are commonplace in the good book.

Once an individual receives a degree or designation in one of the modalities that constitutes what natural healing is all about, this achievement only opens up the door to more learning. Most knowledgeable or "proven" therapies are discovered through in-the-field trial and error, or professional experience.

Once a particular path or course is chosen, only then can one begin the necessary research and study commitment required, in order to afford the degreed individual an opportunity and challenge to rise to that status known as a qualified practitioner.

In my own journey and thirst to seek more knowledge in my field of expertise, I continued my quest for learning led to including a place for my

Resource Reference Library. It includes the best of advice as offered by recognized PhDs sharing similar specialties as my own. Those are practitioners well known for their knowledge and achievements through in-the-field efforts and achievements. Annually that could be an investment of hundreds of dollars, but an investment well worth the dollars spent. Not only are these books often referred to, but also they can sometimes be the second opinion that I might appreciate. These practitioners have paid their dues, put their time in and earned the respect of public and peers.

As they willingly passed down their wisdom, I have been grateful to be able to incorporate a bit of their wisdom in with my own. The library as grown and includes books and information from biochemists, naturopaths, nutritionists and herbalists.

Herbalists and N.D.'S who advocate natural healing (including many medical doctors) often believe in and support the idea of (as communicated to their patients) taking advantage of all beneficial alternatives available, especially those that are inline with one's belief system.

With time and experience under my belt I grew in understanding through listening to all who came seeking my help, and in hearing what each has said has taught me. For in sharing in which recommendations really worked for them, as well as hearing what others have pointed to as providing little benefit, I have learned. As I continue to uncover facts regarding the remarkable non-toxic remedies that I have long believed in, and ascribed to, I am in awe of their remarkable qualities! Yet these remedies and the practitioners who have studied them are not yet fully utilized by the overall populations. This may be due in part, because many have little knowledge regarding these therapies, as well as there being few skilled available practitioners in many geographic areas.

In fact, many Insurers impede the ability for practitioners to effectively practice their skills. For example, when Renders Wellness was founded in 1995, it was very difficult to secure adequate professional liability insurance.

Therefore, I plunged right in and had some hurdles to overcome even before using the skills I was trained for. I found that the type of opposition that is born out of ignorance was a hurdle that many professionals before me had also to overcome, including the medical establishment.

Without having witnessed firsthand how many of these wonderful herbs could be beneficial to patients (minus side-effects that are associated with many drugs used to treat the same disorder), I soon realized that I had come into my own time.

As long as I could see the positive effects derived through the professional use of concentrated nutrients (including herbs), I would continue to believe in what it was I had been pursuing.

It was about that same time that it also became evident to me that what I had learned would become meaningless without having an opportunity to teach and share that knowledge with others. Perhaps it is just this philosophy that has carried many religions down through the centuries, learning and sharing! For love is not passive and requires action! Suffice it to say then, Love and Sharing is a phenomenon in which the more we give away, the more we are renewed!

****

One

Alternative Medicine Opportunity

On March 16, 1996 a local newspaper ran a story title: Nature's Alternative Treatments aid HIV-positive patients. The article went on to relay how the Federal government was funding a program for the HIV/AIDS that included such Alternative therapies as: Acupuncture, Herbal and Vitamin therapies, Chiropractic care and biofeedback.

At the time the Story was released, the program had already been underway in the Spanish Community Center in the Wildwood, New Jersey area, and was funding such treatments for more than 200 HIV/AIDS individuals at a cost of $37,000.00.

Although it seemed somewhat odd at the time that federal money was paying for herbs such as Milk thistle and Cat's claw, people using the services were voicing opinions expressing how they felt these remedies in some instances, to be lifesavers.

The money for these Alternative therapies had come from the federal Ryan White Care Act, which Congress had not yet renewed and which soon could be cut. While some pondered whether this funding would be cut, many HIV/AIDS individuals were praying that it would not be cut. These individuals were claiming how Alternative therapies had given them hope, and yet another day without pain.

1

In 1996 the New Jersey grant (program) was continued, this time however under the supervision of The Atlantic City Medical center's HIV Consortium.

While names have been changed to protect the privacy of many individuals diagnosed with HIV, their comments were heard and their cries for the program to continue were answered. Steve (while this is not his real name, we'll call him Steve) was one of those HIV-positive individuals who had been diagnosed five years earlier in 1991.

For about a year he took AZT (an abbreviation for the long named drug used to treat the HIV/AIDS populations. Yet Steve continually complained about side effects from the drug to his doctor, only to leave his doctor's office again and again without solutions, or an alternative. However since beginning the program as a new applicant, and being provided recommendations from Renders Wellness that were being paid for through the new Ryan White Funding program, Steve claimed that he was feeling much better. This led to Steve adopting a more positive attitude. The whole idea of these treatments, according to Steve, was exactly what he had been looking for. According to Steve (and I had to agree with him) his disease was all about the immune system. Many patients were realizing that if they could build up their immune system, they would be in a much better position for inhibiting replication of the virus and preventing AIDS. These herbs and vitamins according to Steve, did not produce any side effects and did not therefore, lead to more medication for addressing side effects such as had been the custom up until this point.

Steve's own story is not unique however, and there was a growing consensus among many of the HIV that this new approach to treating HIV really did work and was non-toxic!

To quote The Atlantic City Press newspapers own remarks: "Clearly it is recognized at the federal level that these are alternatives to your standard medical approaches to treatment of HIV and AIDS." A program manager stated that it all started as a reaction to the inability of traditional medicine to address some of the problems that surround HIV and AIDS. Carmen Grasso (the then, Program Manager) also stated that while medicine's ability to fight the virus has improved, natural approaches are being given more credence. These therapies he continued, are not being pushed at the expense of medical or traditional treatments. His words confirmed once again that these therapies (nutritional and herbal) are being utilized and paid for only because they were found in clinical trials to be effective!

One HIV patient discussed how he had been using vitamins and herbs therapeutically long before hearing about the development of this program, but was happy that he would be eligible for coverage as it often cost him as much as $200.00 to $300.00 per month for his vitamins and herbs. A cost however, that the new program would now be able to help with. Another woman we will refer to as Diane (No real names will be used) from Atlantic County relayed to Renders Wellness how she was disgusted (her words) with traditional medicine because for her it caused rashes,

3

insomnia and many other annoying side effects. Diane had been searching for some time, hoping to find an alternative treatment.

****

TWO

N.I.H. (National Institutes of Health) Study gives legitimacy to Alternative Medicine

In March of 1996 the Press of Atlantic City newspaper carried an article stating that the National Institutes of Health with its traditional conservative views (and an advocate to conservative medicine) now has an office specifically for Alternative Medicine. It went on to say that the office soon would be funding a $1 million study of alternative medicines for the supportive treatment of HIV-positive individuals.

The study itself was being conducted by Bastyr University in Seattle. And while it was too early to guess at the results, it was apparent that its mere existence would lend legitimacy to alternative medicine. A therapy that many people in the HIV-positive community have been calling for. This decision resulted from a five-year study into alternative therapies as to whether or not; they could be beneficial to the HIV population. At the end of this five-year study, the results were conclusive. The specialties that showed the most benefit were: Nutrition, Chiropractic services, Herbal remedies, Massage therapy and Stress reduction exercises.

Cherie Reeves, the project's coordinator, said the study was looking at 178 treatments and medicines, including Acupuncture, traditional Chinese medicine, homeopathic and naturopathic medicine, massage therapy and many types of herbs.

5

However, Reeves said the two-year study is anecdotal, not clinical. Meaning it would rely on patients to report their progress, rather than more scientific methods such as double-blind studies.

Still Reeves however, affirmed how the study could only prove to be valuable. "Research hasn't been done on alternative medicine," she explained because: "Funding hasn't been available."

Alternative medicine's role in fighting cancer and other diseases is also being studied at other colleges across the country.

"There are many people who believe alternative medicine provides additional care and treatment for HIV-positive populations" said Reeves. "But" she added: "Many believe it will take a lot of study to confirm or disprove those suspicions."

Bastyr was actively looking for people to participate in their study.

THREE

Renders Wellness is sub-contracted by the Atlantic City Medical Center's HIV CONSORTIUM to provide services in Naturopathy.

It had been decided that the funding would be made available to individuals only in those cities where the highest rate of diagnosed HIV had been reported. Consequently, Atlantic City became one of those cities approved for the program. This new funding was to be managed in Atlantic City through The Atlantic City Medical Center's HIV Consortium, as part of The Ryan White Fund distributed through The National Institutes of Health in Bethesda, MD.

When we, at Renders Wellness became aware of this new funding program for the HIV/AIDS population in our area, we immediately made application to be accepted as a sub-contractor through The Atlantic City Medical center's HIV Consortium. Soon afterward, we were accepted and were asked to provide nutritional support, herbal remedies and guided imagery for the HIV/AIDS population of two counties: Atlantic County and Cape May County.

However as time passed and other individuals and organizations from nearby communities learned about the program, Renders Wellness soon found that we

7

was doing a bit more traveling. Although the program only paid for recommendations for those qualified individuals from the two specified counties, other HIV Support groups only looked for the information and recommendations we were able to provide them with. They were willing to fund their own supplements. The Catholic Charity was definitely doing their part by remaining involved.

Many of the participants in the program became eligible only if they met the criteria requirements as set up by the program. Requirements included that each applicant not exceed a pre-determined scale for maximum income. This program was instituted in order to provide support for those individuals whose income did not provide them freedom to neither explore choices, nor experiment with options such as massage therapy or guided imagery. Applicants with minimum income according to the pre-determined scale, or those with inadequate medical insurance coverage were readily accepted into the program. Often many of the applicants were unemployed due to health problems. Without a steady income, most were left without a car, or transportation.

Therefore the HIV Management team often required Renders Wellness to travel between several locations in the Atlantic City and Cape May area. Appointments were carried out at a specified county building.

Our first implementation when meeting with new clients was to do a complete intake. That included date of diagnosis, current meds and prognosis. We also included a Disclosure as required by our Insurance carrier that clearly spelled out our credentials and what our services included.

As a sub-contractor for the HIV Consortium our role was to guide these patients through relaxation exercises into a state where stress could be alleviated. Many of these newly diagnosed HIV patients were dealing with many issues. They were dealing with their own vulnerability, uncertainty about their future, drug addiction, financial problems and family acceptance of the disease. Often times, in revealing their newly diagnosed disease to a family member might mean a first time acknowledgement to a loved one of a drug addiction, promiscuity or homosexuality.

Therefore, it was easily understood how being newly diagnosed with HIV or AIDS could lead to a high level of stress. Stress however, could become instrumental in further contributing to an escalation of the progression of the disease. Guided Imagery was a time wherein each interested participant could spend forty-five minutes to an hour of learning how to shut out the world and retreat to a quiet, peaceful world within themselves.

Once this experience is felt, motivation for learning and practicing this technique again and again is created. In managing one's stress level, each individual is better able to think more clearly, accept their diagnosis without associating it with a death sentence, and be more open and ready to learning strategies that will not only lengthen their lives, but enhance the very quality of their lives.

FOUR

How Renders Wellness Created And Implemented the HIV/AIDS Protocol

At the same time we did our intake, we had each patient sign off on an Authorization form allowing us to contact their respective physicians at The Infectious Disease Center. While Renders Wellness Began by collecting all relative data on each patient through their medical physician, other goals were instituted. One primary goal was to research the disease as far as we could, in order to better understand the progression of the disease, and what conditions might be associated with the progression of HIV/AIDS virus.

Part of that would include understanding and interpreting blood test results that were markers for stability and/or progression of the disease.

Each participant opting to include nutrition and herbal recommendations as part of their support system in management of the disease came to Renders Wellness and were given two sets of recommendations: General recommendations (including compounds best avoided ~ antagonists and toxins), including healthier replacements for these denatured foods, or prescriptions for common symptoms such as: Insomnia, nausea, headache and other secondary problems. Then they were given specific recommendations (herbs and nutrients) that

10

were meant to detoxify the liver, correct deficiencies and enhance the immune system.

Some recommendations were provided in order to eliminate the necessity for prescribing yet another medication for handling the side effects associated with potent cocktails such as AZT, and for the purpose of enhancing the immune system. This was essential in order to understand how involvement in their health care was essential. For instance, in eliminating the number of drugs being taken, as well as the potency of these drugs could often help in the detoxification process of the liver. Also, the ability to be able to decrease the frequency in which these potent drugs were taken could also have a positive effect on their immune system. In other words, their involvement was essential for empowerment and encouraged. Involvement in managing of a disease helps to alleviate feelings of hopelessness that often exists in

Individuals understood, or were soon encouraged many such individuals. Studies have shown that our very attitude, or emotions can have either a positive, or negative effect upon our being, including the immune system.

By decreasing the number of toxins that these patients were ingesting, we were effectively supporting the liver and the burden often placed upon the liver as a result of the taking many of these prescribed and potent drugs for extended periods.

While it is true that the kidneys often are involved in the detoxifying process, and often assist in the removal of toxins from the body, the liver is the key component responsible for filtering out of toxins from the body. As we have learned, whenever the body's filtering organs are over-stressed for an extended period of time, there is what is known as an "Accumulative effect"! When this event gradually begins to occur, the immune system is further compromised due to an inadequate elimination of toxins.

This is exactly what we work to prevent through nutritional support, detoxification and stimulation of the immune system through natural remedies, an attempt to prevent HIV from advancing into AIDS due to a gradual weakening of the body's natural resources. In the most vulnerable state, HIV replication advances thereby overcoming the weakened immune system. Our best weapon against any disease is to understand the enemy and to take charge in areas where we can exert a positive change. Naturally (not meant to be a pun), we took the extra time, went the extra mile to educate each and every HIV/AIDS individual we came into contact with. Education often goes hand in hand with motivation, another essential element in the war against HIV. Because HIV is an immune disorder, it is imperative to avoid more toxins that weaken the immune response and to work toward enhancement of the immune system.

Naturopathy employs the benefits of all non-toxic remedies, including concentrated nutrients. These supplements and recommendations are non-addictive, and non-toxic!

With each initial Consultation, the referred patient is required to sign a disclaimer-confirming acknowledgement in having been informed that Renders Wellness does not examine, diagnose, prescribe drugs, nor promise cures! Furthermore, the disclaimer states that each participant in the program is responsible for advising their respective physicians of any protocols recommended to them by Renders Wellness. In that way, they are able to ask questions and discuss concerns with their physician. Whenever a physician requests a copy of our recommendations, we immediately comply.

Communication between practitioners is encouraged. It is important that each be aware of any possible contraindications in order to make the best recommendations available for each individual. Initial Consultations also included a newly devised set of general instructions for each new participant such as taking a good "One A Day" multiple vitamins.

We also provided them with a partial list of denatured and devitalized foods that were to be avoided such as alcohol, cigarettes, refined white sugar (an acid), hydrogenated oils (suspected carcinogens) often found in junk foods and/or fried foods. With the legal aspects of our new project, as well as the general specifics taken care of, we turned our attention toward the task of research, compilation, review and selection of those nutrients and herbs determined to be most beneficial through clinical trials. Beneficial that is, without having any side effects associated with them. Time and attention was given to our goal of effectively being able to lower the number of drugs being taken into the body, as well as the potency and frequency of them. This, we believed at Renders Wellness would alleviate the burden placed upon the liver, or its ability to filter out toxic residues often left behind as a result of aggressive drug therapy.

With our new contract in hand, and our priorities in mind, we set about preparing necessary copies and leaflets for hand outs, and soon began a series of Lectures that were held at Hospitals, Charity Organizations and of course, Infectious Disease Centers.

FIVE

Immediate Problematic Findings

As we began to see patients that were referred to us from The Atlantic City Medical center's HIV Consortium, we soon began to see an area where we could be of most help. That, we believed, would be through the lowering of the patient's toxic load. These patients were diagnosed at the Hospital, but were in fact being medically treated at a couple of local Infectious Disease Centers. Our immediate determination was an over-whelming sense of ability to lessen the toxic load by making recommendations to replace potent drugs that were being prescribed to alleviate the side effects caused by the initial drugs being prescribed to treat the HIV virus.

Many of these potent drugs not only placed a huge burden on the body's Liver, but came with a whole new set of intolerable symptoms that were being addressed with yet another whole new set of drugs. Often times, we were actually able to see the result of this toxic overload in the swelling of the Liver that was quite visible to the naked eye.

Patients often described themselves as being more intolerable with regard to dealing with the side effects associated with the medications they were being prescribed than with the actual symptoms of the disease! These side effects had a whole range of emotional and spiritual effects upon many of the patients we met in a clinical setting and this was confirmed by their own words.

In a private setting without any feeling of haste, most of these HIV individuals often felt a need to confide their inner most personal feelings about their new diagnosis to a trusted practitioner. They felt safe, as there was no emotional attachment. Some relayed a feeling they perceived as punished from God for having used drugs, participating in a promiscuous life style, or homosexual behavior. Often however, when they were able to think things through sufficiently, or spend some quiet time talking to their Creator, they were able to let go of many of these feelings that dampened their will to survive! This is always a positive first step into therapy.

Many came to understand that it was their own choices and life style that had put them in harm's way, and not God's will to punish. In fact, they soon realized that God loved them and that HIV/AIDS was not necessarily a death sentence. Once again, they now had choices regarding their life and their future!

Unfortunately, many ignorant people contribute to the burden placed upon the HIV population, many unknowingly! This is due to a mindset that leaves little room for compassion, and is born out of ignorance!

This type of thinking has always been at the center of discrimination. And this lack of empathy from a minority still contributes today to adding to the burden that the HIV must bear. Ironically, often times it is those very individuals who are guilty of this type of discrimination and persecution who call themselves children of God. The Righteous! To most of us however, God *is* love and love is healing.

A loving God created all of us, and it is my personal belief that He will lead us all if we allow Him. However, most of us do not see God as an authoritarian who takes to whipping off His belt strap in order to "Teach us a lesson" as many would have us believe!

An individual with HIV/AIDS is not necessarily gay or an intravenous drug user, nor can any of us assume that they are practicing indiscriminate sex with a multitude of partners.

In this day and age we now understand that many innocent individuals contract HIV through tainted blood while receiving a blood transfusion. Little babies are an example of just how the innocent too can become infected. Hundreds of children are born each year to parents where at least one of them are HIV, and have knowingly, or unknowingly infected their offspring.

While it may be true that many HIV positive individuals were infected by dirty needles and as a result of being a drug user, and others may have become HIV because they sold their bodies for money, we do not know the circumstances of what led them down such a path. And we certainly have not been appointed judge and jury!

17

Let me share with you a beautiful story about a young woman who ended up in Calcutta, India immediately following a divorce. She decided to spend two weeks there offering her services to the needy through the Charity Order founded by Mother Therese, now Blessed Saint Therese. While the young woman worked professionally as a Beautician, she wanted to help in any way that she could help the poor.

The young woman was confident that while she worked in a positive way helping others, she would be able to clear her head and find peace and direction in her life!

When she finally found herself on the doorstep of the Charity Center, she suddenly became conscious of her attire. Standing there in a somewhat brief skirt with stockings and high heels, she was embarrassed knowing that her attire was inappropriate. Meekly she knocked on the door and sheepishly smiled when the petite nun answered her knock. The friendly nun seemed to be expecting the weary traveler and gave her a wide smile, waving her inside. After a snack, the nun showed her to her room and told her to rest.

The next day, the very same nun whom we shall call Sister Mary came to collect her guest and take her to the Convalescent Center where she would begin her volunteer work. It is a place where many of the poor, elderly and homeless were housed.

Sister Mary directed the young woman toward a bed where an elderly woman lay quietly. She looked quite frail, and her clothing was tattered and worn. The young woman was somewhat taken back by the looks and the smell that emanated from the old woman's bed.

The Nun instructed the young woman to take the old woman to a small alcove area across the room where there was a sink and a table with soap and clean towels. There she was to bath the elderly lady. The young woman (whom we will now refer to as Ellen) looked again at the elderly woman and then back again at Sister Mary blurting out: "Sister I am sorry, but I cannot possibly do this! Is there something else I can do instead Sister?" The nun's eyes twinkled as she smiled at Ellen when she answered saying, "That's alright, do not worry about it, I'll do it." The nun went to the bed of the frail old woman as she literally lifted her with both hands under her body and carried her to the other side of the room. There in the alcove, Sister Mary began to bathe the old woman. Ellen followed the nun and helplessly watched from a distance. That part of the room was small and sort of darkened as there was only one small window in the center that was higher than the women themselves.

However, as Sister Mary cradled the old woman across her lap, holding onto her with her left hand under her back, with her right hand she began to wash the old lady with a tenderness that Ellen had never seen before. Suddenly as Ellen continued to watch, she became witness to a gradual illumination from the small overhead window as it outlined the pair of women like a halo.

Ellen was transfixed as she watched the nun bathe the elderly woman who was draped across her lap. What Ellen saw is a sight that remains with her today.

19

For the body that lay across the lap of the small nun began to resemble the body of Christ after He had been taken down from the cross (The Pieta). Sister Mary in her gown and cloak with her head bent in tenderness became the vision of Jesus' mother. Ellen was overcome with awe and the tears began to flow, and her mind was soon filled with words from the bible she had once heard that seemed very apropos for the setting. The words that Ellen heard in her heart now were these words said by Christ: "Whatever you do for the least of My brethren, you do for Me!"

From that day forward Ellen's life was changed forever. She gladly began to throw herself into the many chores that were offered to her.

Before the young woman left the Center at the end of the month, she spoke to the Sister Mary again asking for her guidance. "How can I help others Sister as a Beautician, it seems to be such a superficial job now after having spent time here in Calcutta?" Once again sister smiled and said: "There are many people dear who have been maimed through birth defects, or accidents who do not feel good about themselves. Perhaps you could help them with their Make-up, and more than that, you might reach them where it hurts and let them feel the love that is inside you, the love that is God's gift to you."

Ellen had learned a lot in just two short weeks in that convent helping others who were less fortunate than she. Magically or mystically, whenever she was busy helping others, Ellen forgot about her own problems. The reward? She found direction, peace, satisfaction and meaning in her life. She had received more than she had hoped for.

Working with the HIV and AIDS individuals for nearly three years in three separate counties, it soon became evident to me that the HIV population is much like the rest of us. While some it is true, may have made a couple of poor choices in life, which of us has not been there, or done that? All the more reason they needed to feel loved and accepted.

Never before could there ever have been a better example of Holistic medicine at work than in this new program, which encompassed the essence of body, mind and spirit! Total healing does not, nor should not exclude the human spirit. Indeed I was grateful to have been called to the challenge, and Renders Wellness accepted that challenge with eagerness.

SIX

Initial Intake Interviews

As a N. D. or Doctor of Naturopathy, I felt as though I had somehow finally reached that place in life where I not only wanted to be, but where I truly felt I was being led by the God of my understanding.

Though my practice is small, it lends itself well to soothing the spirit and touching the soul! Situated on nearly four wooded acres that has a small stream that runs along its border, it is by every sense of the word, pristine. Untouched by man. Other than our home and attached office Suite with a private entrance, our home is a two story, recently remodeled cedar shake building of approximately 3,000 square feet. The office itself is a glass solarium that overlooks the woods and the dozens of handmade birdhouses that are replenished every day with bird food, making it a home for many exotic birds. On any given day, one might see a cardinal, blue jay, dove, wren, chickadee, wild finch, rabbit, and even a hawk. Chipmunks are often seen playing together. Early in the morning one might encounter a deer grazing in the back yard, or hear the cries of a Fox at night.

Many are surprised by the fact that such a property exists just a couple of miles from the busy Somers Point area, or the beaches of Ocean City, N.J.

Because my own life is full of peace and serenity, in part due to the work that I do and a good marriage, I am able to impart that message in my demeanor. The environment in which Renders Wellness sits of course, also imparts that message of tranquility! Often, a Guided Imagery client has told us that it is more than the Guided Imagery session that brings them a sense of peace before leaving Renders Wellness.

These messages are affirmation that I am doing the right thing with my time and my life! But of course, have briefcase and will travel was a part of what we did back in those days, whenever the situation necessitated. At the end of each session it became customary too, to say goodbye with a hug! A hug is a good way to relieve tension or stress, and a good way of expressing sincerity! Before each new individual left the office, they received a Relaxation tape to take with him/her to be used again at home.

Often, perhaps it was the setting itself that triggered an opening up of the private world of many HIV that came through our office doors. It was as though they needed to break down the walls that had long ago become barriers that surrounded their hearts.

They were feeling comfortable and showed their trust in me. It had been always our custom to spend a minimum of 45 minutes to an hour with each client. It was our goal to insure that no one would ever feel rushed as though they were simply a name, or a number. That is a practice that is still carried out today. It is my belief that good feelings stimulate the release of good bio-chemicals, and raise optimism and motivation. The result is a more optimum functioning Immune system. And which of us could live without hope?

We were on a first name basis, many of my clients and myself. The atmosphere was always comfortable, however conversation always remained very professional. While it is my custom as a professional to avoid the pitfall of turning a patient into a personal friend, when they were in my office there was no one else in the world more important to me than them.

Each individual and their privacy (including their personal stories) are sworn to professional secrecy and a personal code of ethics. However, some of the backgrounds were so touching that I'd like to share a few of their stories here with you now. Of course, names, addresses and any information that might identify an individual will be changed in order to protect the party.

SEVEN

Case Histories
Case #1 ~ Cassie
Cassie and Bill:

Cassie (not her real name) was a woman of about 29 years of age when first we met. Cassie was bordering on full-blown Aids! However, she did not appear depressed and showed no sign of self-pity. Cassie made no apologies for who she was, and proudly exuded a genuine air of confidence. She expressed herself as a woman with quite a bit of spunk and often teasingly, with a quality she referred to as *attitude!* Yet she openly embraced me as though I had been a long lost friend!

She was easy to like, and while she had a lot to live for, Cassie was not accustomed to taking direction very well. If there was anything at all that Cassie might have lacked, one might say that it was consistency. Perhaps this was never more noticeable than when it came to following her daily regimen. Often she'd fall back into smoking cigarettes as they were familiar and Cassie enjoyed all that she became fond of. She seemed to have a strong resistance to letting go of anything she truly enjoyed! Running out of her recommendations due to neglect, or maybe a lack of money contributed to her final breakdown.

However, I suspected that Cassie had really never mastered much control in her life. She confided how

25

she had always been a people pleaser. A bit late perhaps (but one could argue that fact), Cassie revealed how she came to realize that just maybe, she had put herself last too often. She pondered deeply, perhaps thinking maybe, could it be that Cassie believed that she was not deserving of true happiness? Cassie often relayed how she did not feel deserving of such a loving partner as she now had in her life!

It was not unusual for her partner in life, Bill to accompany Cassie to my office for her scheduled visit. While Cassie did not have a car and lived in Atlantic City, which is about seventeen miles from my office (where transportation to my office is not convenient), Cassie still insisted on meeting me on my own turf, rather than allowing me to make the trip out to her. It mattered not to her that I had been making regular trips out her way for others, and would continue to do so. That was Cassie!

On one particular occasion when Bill was with Cassie at our office, I could not help but notice Bill's attentiveness to Cassie, and his sincere concern for her. Just to acknowledge the good qualities I noticed in there relationship, I asked: "How did you two meet?" There was a pause; a moment of silence and then that silence was broken by Cassie's laughter. It resonated throughout the entire building. Still, it was Cassie who was the first to speak up saying: "Bill was one of my Tricks." Bill laughed too, and for a moment, I knew that my face had turned crimson. It was not Cassie's previous method of earning money that shocked me, but it was the fact that this man who loved her so dearly was able to *not* judge her for that! Even more,

26

what struck me most was not so much as how the two of them had gotten together, but how Bill who was not HIV was able to put his own life on the line in order to be with the woman he loved.

Let me follow up by adding to that by saying, to the best of my knowledge, Bill was not, nor ever had he been a drug user. He worked every day to make a living for the two of them. I say this with confidence because as I knew the two of them, honesty was a part of what held them together. This I had found to be consistent with most HIV diagnosed individuals. If ever there was a time for reality and honesty, you might say this was it!

Just to imagine that kind of giving of one's self is much more than I would have anticipated in coming from many of us. While I was the teacher who provided health information, I was learning much about life! Bill made it his responsibility (knowing Cassie all too well) to not only pay for many of Cassie's supplements and herbs that were not covered in the program, but to insure that she took them in a timely fashion! He drove her to many of her Consultation visits, and never deserted her because of her diagnosis.

Openness, unselfishness, humility and willingness to easily love were insights that I had gratefully been given through my work with the poor and the afflicted.

Although by comparison my own life seemed fulfilling and was blessed with many gifts, including this new sense of achievement, I was still able to learn and take lessons from others. With each new day, more

27

and more, I felt that I was truly grasping much of what I understood to be the real meaning of life!

The last time I saw Cassie she looked to be about five months pregnant. She was not of course, and it soon became obvious that her liver was inflamed and she was in toxic overload!

Note: Renders Wellness declined the offer to participate after the third year in the program because the program had made severe cutbacks. In their new revision, it was decided that each new HIV/AIDS (or those already in the program) would be allowed only one Consultation at Renders Wellness. Realizing that one visit could be about as beneficial to each participant as one vitamin, or one meal, we saw that the only right thing to do would be to verbalize as much to the committee, before leaving the program.

Case History #2 ~ Johnny

Johnny lived in a bordering county not covered by the Ryan White funding program, yet he had heard about the program and called our office to schedule a visit. Johnny lived with his mother and was about 40 years of age. Obviously nervous and looking very sad, Johnny confided he was felt desperate! He had been in and out of the Hospital with upper respiratory problems, pneumonia, and recurrent Candida infections. He expressed a desire and willingness to being involved with nutritional support and herbal recommendations. He had been prescribed and was taking a powerful drug known as AZT. In combination with a couple of other drugs, it was known as a *Cocktail.* Information on AZT will be found in another chapter along with other medical drugs often prescribed in the treatment of HIV/AIDS.

Johnny felt hopeless and feared that at his age he had little to look forward to as far as a cure was concerned. Though he remained faithful to the taking of his prescribed medications, he was concerned because they had not prevented him from getting ill and/or being hospitalized time and again.

A gifted pianist, Johnny sent me a small crocheted angel and a recorded tape of him playing a Christmas carol on his organ. Johnny soon gave up his fight with each new hospital admission, and his stress level continued to climb. Johnny vacillated with regard to his feelings and wishes as to a preferred form of treatment.

After awhile Johnny just dropped out of sight, and we are not certain where Johnny is today! While we had not seen Johnny at our office for more than just a couple of visits, his gift of the little crocheted angel still sits on a shelf in my office.

Tracking of patients was not part of our service; therefore we respected each individual's right to privacy and did not make any attempt to reconstitute therapy. It is we believe, only beneficial when therapy is entered into freely with hope and anticipation!

Without an inner belief, or hope in one's future, one would have no commitment and therefore, would not remain faithful to the program. Sadly, confidence and hope seemed to be lacking in Johnny's demeanor.

Case History #3 ~ Lavonia

Lavonia was a divorced woman of approximately 39 years of age. She had a couple of older children who were out on their own. Lavonia lived in the next county South of Atlantic County and shared a home with a female partner.

She was an attractive woman who with a couple of breaks could have been successful in just about anything she might have endeavored. Lavonia was at peace with herself and her life as it was, and with her partner. She smiled a lot and was a very warm and friendly soul. With Lavonia, I felt as though I had known her for years. She was that comfortable to be around.

Also, with Lavonia as with most of the others, she did not blame anyone for her unfortunate circumstances, nor was she in any way down on life! Instead, she took each day in stride. Staying on the positive side, Lavonia was grateful for whatever helps and/or friendship was extended to her.

Able to greatly reduce the number of drugs Lavonia was taking through stress reduction, nutritional support and immune enhancement, she was soon able to reduce the toxic load and gain some control over her disease. An ideal situation for reducing the potential for going into full-blown AIDS. Eventually Lavonia and her partner made a geographical move and that was the last we saw of her.

Case History #4 ~ Tim and Ralph

Tim and Ralph were two young men who came to Renders Wellness just two weeks after having tested positive for HIV. They were so nervous and depressed that it was difficult for either one of them to remain seated for as long as it took to complete the Interview. Each wanted to be seen and treated together as a couple.

Ironically, their new diagnosis seemed to bring them much closer. They were bound to one another in life and in sex, and now it appeared that they planned on facing death together!

And it was as though it was death that each felt they had been sentenced to. In conversation, each expressed a similar belief saying: (and I quote them) "*God* is punishing us for living this gay lifestyle!" Because they were gay! They bought into that small mindedness and were therefore, inconsolable! They talked about going home and facing their respective parents with not only the news that they were gay (a fact that had been hidden from family up until this point), but now diagnosed HIV. They expressed feelings of fear and emotions that ran from guilt to remorse!

In most instances, emotional counseling is necessary. Counseling is required not only that individuals begin to feel better about themselves and accept their diagnosis, but stress and negative feelings further burden the immune response!

These young men were obviously not yet ready to begin focusing in on how they planned to manage and treat their disorder, they appeared to be temporarily more intent on coming to terms with their disease, sharing with their parents and other members of their families, before they could move on and focus in on themselves.

They looked at me in this their moment of change as a turning point in their lives and an opportunity to confirm their willingness to make amends to God and change their lifestyle. They vowed that they would return to their respective faiths and live a healthier lifestyle. Their words, not mine! While I was not trained professionally to counsel these young men either emotionally or spiritually, I did make it a point to offer them the idea that their new diagnosis was not necessarily a punishment from God, nor a death sentence, but was a sexually transmitted disease.

Still, they chanted on about how they felt that if they had lived a cleaner life, God would love and accept them. If ever it could be said that out of darkness comes the Light, these two young men had gone through a tremendous transition in just a couple of weeks, and I was their Confessor!

They showed a sincere desire to share how they now could see how their partying days and selfishness (all for the sake of fun and instant gratification) had been nothing but evil. They seemed to be saying that while temptations exist in life for all of us, if we were wise we would turn away.

Although these two young men were not even close to 30, they were internally feeling their vulnerability and looking death square in the face. Now they wanted nothing more than to return to God where they felt they would be safe and loved and protected! It was obvious to me how the last two weeks for these young men had taken them on a journey to hell and back again.

On top of all of that, here they were telling all to a middle aged Doctor of Natural healing. Immediately, recommendations for non-toxic, non-addictive herbs and supplements were provided to help calm the nervous system, and support the immune system.

Of course it had to be said that these young men, much like the rest of us would one day die, that is true! But who of us could predict when? With the right care and attitude, God willing, they might not cross that threshold until each had reached a ripe old age. Only God knows the day or the hour.

Still I reaffirmed to them that theirs was a manageable disease and that their diagnosis was not a reflection of God's wrath! It was further explained to them how with a somewhat more conservative lifestyle, together with a healthier nutritional program (including a few herbal immune boosters), they very well might enjoy a relatively normal life.

After a few more tears, Tim and Ralph soon began to realize that regardless of what that little piece of white paper they held in their hand read, life must go on. And I reminded them that in time, thoughts of HIV would no longer dominate their every thought!

These young men eventually returned home to their respective families in one of the Southern States and that was the last we heard, or saw of them.

****

Case Histories 5, 6 & 7 ~

How could I ever forget the individuals who quite frankly were already into full-blown AIDS when first we met? Because their time was divided into constantly being readmitted and released from the hospital, to continually visiting their primary care physician for follow-up care, it was next to impossible unfortunately, to provide much support. While HIV is often manageable and without excessive toxicity effect upon the liver, AIDS on the other hand, often places the patient in a position were detoxification is next to impossible. This is because the liver is already experiencing a high level of toxicity due to the high does of potent cocktails they are taking.

The greatest benefit or effect of natural remedies upon the HIV individual is attained *before* HIV progresses into AIDS. In full blown AIDS the body is already operating through the mechanical aid of drugs, rather than through its own biochemistry. In other words, the liver has already reached a high level of toxicity, which contributes to the progression of the disease. When the liver itself is no longer functioning properly, it will become inflamed and that swelling is often visible to the naked eye! At this point, it is often too late for detoxification, or for stimulating the natural immune response.

Case History #8 ~ Don

Don (all names are fictitious) was a young man who had a lot to live for. When first I met Don he was eager to tell me his story. A married man with two young children, Don had once been a very accomplished athlete, a Swimmer.

He had broken his neck in a Swimming accident, and at some point was given a transfusion of blood that was tainted. Don soon afterward, became infected with the HIV virus. For whatever reason, Don was separated and going through a divorce. Don had suddenly gone from being an athlete with a family to an invalid out of work and flat on his back with HIV.

Talk about your tough breaks! Don thrived however, on his two young children, a boy of about 10 and a girl of about 8. Often they were with him on an extended visit, and Don had an Aunt or family member who came in a couple of times a day to feed him and check on him. It was obvious upon driving up to the house and parking the car that soon the house he called home would be gone too. Or there on the front lawn loomed a formidable Sale sign.

His children were there with him the first time I arrived, and actually wanted to partake in the Guided Imagery session with their dad. They did not giggle as children might be expected to do, but found themselves dreamy and sleepy by the end of the session. Don laughed. His eyes lit up when he looked at them, or spoke about them. It was obvious that they were his life, and brought him great joy and pride!

Don found much peace and energy through Visualization and Meditation exercises. Renders wellness had created several audiotapes for listening, including recommendations for digestion and metabolism. As always, we would leave behind guided imagery tapes. Don had a problem in both swallowing and digesting due to his Swimming accident, which led to his broken neck. And for the most part, lay totally immobile. Don told me that whenever he was alone and able to listen to a tape, it helped him to visualize being somewhere else and doing something that he loved. This was accomplishing then, the task it was meant to do, to help Don to relax.

Due to Don's problem with swallowing, many of his supplements were provided in a spray container. While Don was in the full-blown Aids stage of his disease, we were able only to assist him in small ways. Progression had taken over at that point, and reversing the progression of this disease is very challenging! Especially, when so many medications are being introduced into a body that is already on toxic overload! Without being a Medical doctor, it was never my custom or intent to suggest anything other than what their primary physician had recommended.

Obviously due to Don's extensive physical injuries, he was unable to exercise and this was a devastating blow to Don. In and out of the hospital with upper respiratory problems, Don would soon be making a geographical change due to the pending sale of his home.

When the day arrived, Don moved out of the area and like many others, we were unable to track his condition. His prognosis however, was not favorable.

****

Case History #9 ~ Bernie

Bernie is a man who came to us from the Program at Atlantic City Medical Center and was diagnosed HIV in about 1987 or 1988. Bernie at that time was 34 to 35 years of age.

Not unlike many of his contemporaries, being a black man Bernie took *naturally* (no pun intended) to a Program that was all about concentrated nutrients and herbs, as he was knowledgeable about such therapies. He was, as he had put it "raised on them."

History tells us that herbal remedies for instance, were the primary therapies used for hundreds of years by many cultures, aside from the white Anglo-Saxon American.

Bernie was quick to point out to me that he could not (and was not willing to) tolerate the side effects he experienced as a result of the drugs he had been taking, especially AZT.

AZT or Zidovudine is an antiviral, anti-HIV drug. It was also the first HIV drug most often prescribed. It has been shown in some studies to reverse transcription (a process necessary for replication of the HIV virus) in the HIV infected individual. This drug is metabolized by the body's liver, and eliminated via the kidneys. However, needless to say, patients with either a liver or kidney disorder should not use it.

Side effects of AZT include: Headaches, hypertension, nausea, diarrhea, muscle weakness and/or insomnia. Yet another problem that Bernie had been dealing, which AZT may have exacerbated is hypertension.

To make matters worse, Bernie is an individual who is hypersensitive to many medications, and confessed to having had all of the above described symptoms, most often associated with the drug AZT.

He came into The Renders Wellness Program with open arms and embraced it! He relayed to us that he would rather die than continue to live on the drug. He was not yet full blown AIDS, and was therefore a good candidate for Natural Therapeutics!

Bernie refused to continue taking the drug, and was willing to go to any lengths in following our recommendations for detoxification, stress reduction, Immune enhancement and nutritional support.

After the usual Intake information and Lab work copies that are customary on one's initial office consultation, we worked with Bernie on his nutritional profile, providing him a list of foods to avoid. However it has always been our belief that when Rules handed down, they are better adhered to when one understands why it is they should follow the rules!

Next, we provided Bernie with healthier replacement foods for those that now topped our list of foods to avoid.

A list of these foods will be found in another Chapter.

Each Client completed a Bio-equilibrium questionnaire that provided us with the necessary information for addressing annoying symptoms, symptoms associated with toxic residues from the drugs, allergic responses, or simply part of their Biochemistry profile!

Finally, we provided recommendations that were meant to keep the immune system operating at the highest level of functioning it was capable of operating at. We always stressed at this point, the importance of maintaining consistency in their protocol in order to reap the maximum achievable benefits!

The Atlantic City Medical Center's HIV Consortium (being funded by the N.I.H. or National Institutes of Health) had set up a Program whereby patients were provided a monthly Allowance or Credit at their local Health Food Store where he/she could pick up the necessary supplements (at this point, Renders Wellness instituted an *RD* with a duplicate copy for our records that was similar to an RX, a form to take to the Health Food Store containing their specific recommendations.)

There is a Chapter provided (see index) listing these supplements (nutritional and herbal). However, *self-treatment* is not advised. Doses are offered only through Consultation for providing maximum benefit, and only after having reviewed and considered all medications being taken by each patient, as well as possible contraindications.

As with any Consultation, client, or disorder there are general recommendations as well as specific recommendations. The general recommendations apply to all, while of course, the specific recommendations target each individual's specific medical diagnosis and prognosis as made by the patient's attending physician. As well as consideration of associated symptoms!

Note: At this time, Bernie had decided (unbeknownst to Renders wellness and/or his primary care physician) to stop all drug medications and concentrate on nutrition, detoxification and immune enhancement through recommendations made by Renders Wellness.

EIGHT

General Recommendations

Prior to taking any individualized, or specific recommendations, it is first necessary to institute the following healthier life-style practices:
To recognize, avoid and eliminate toxins from the body, beginning with the Shopping cart.

What are Toxins?

Toxins are carcinogens, suspected carcinogens and/or antagonists capable of causing a further compromise to the immune system.

What are Antagonists?

Antagonists are substances, chemicals and other compounds that interfere with the body' ability to metabolize, utilize, or store essential nutrients. This can lead to nutritional deficiencies, biochemical imbalances, as well as interfere with optimum functioning of the internal organs that are responsible for the release of proper amounts of hormones, many of which help to protect the immune system. This internal state can cause symptoms that are warnings to the onset of other disorders.

Following is a list of substances that are to be eliminated. In many instances, healthier replacements will be provided.

According to Roberta Altman and Michael J. Sarg, M.D. who is Associate Chief of Medical Oncology St. Vincent's Hospital, New York City and Associate Professor of Clinical Medicine, New York Medical College, and whose book "The Cancer Dictionary" which was called Outstanding for Reference Source for 1993 by the American Library Association. Ms. Altman works for the National Cancer Institute's Cancer Information Service at the Memorial Sloan-Kettering Cancer Center in New York City. A cancer survivor herself, Ms. Altman worked prior to the N.I.H. as an award-winning journalist for NBC Radio as well as Physicians Radio Network.

A partial list:

Carcinogens/Suspected carcinogens

Agent Orange
Arsenic
Artificial Sweeteners Asbestos
Aspartame
Benzenes
Caffeine
Conjugated Equine Estrogen
Decaffeinated coffee
Some drinking water
Electromagnetic fields
Environmental tobacco smoke
Fat
Food Additives

Formaldehyde
Hair dye
Herbicides
Indoor Air Quality
Microwave oven
Mouthwash
Mustard
Nitrites & Nitrates
Nitrosamines
Nuclear Power Plant
Radon
Saccharin
Smoking

Other Suspected Carcinogens

Ultraviolet Radiation
Vinyl Chloride

Pre-cancerous conditions;

Actinic Keratosi
Adenomatous Hyperplasia
Adenomatous Polyps
Adrenal Medullary Tumors
AIDS
Bowen's Disease
Benign Prostatic Hyperplasia
Chronic Atrophic Gastritis
Chronic Ulcerative Colitis
Chronic Vulvar Dystrophy
Chrohn's Disease
Dysplasia
Dysplasia Nevi
Endometrial Hyperplasia
Epstein Barr Virus

Erythoplasia
Genital Herpes Virus
Gonadal Aplasis
Giant Cell Bone Tumor
Human Papilloma Virus
Hyperkeratosis
Intermediate Polyps
Intestinal Metaplasia
Myelodyssplastic Syndrome
Mole
Oldfield's Syndrome
Papilloma Virus
Pernicious Anemia
Plummer-Vinson Syndrome Polyp
Sebaceous Hyperplasia
Sporadic Intestinal Polyps
Turcot's Syndrome
Von Recklinghausen's Neurofibromatosis

Note: More detail is unnecessary, unless one has been diagnosed with any of the above disorders.

Antagonists ~ Compounds, chemicals, or substances when ingested interfere with the body's ability to metabolize, fully utilize, or store essential nutrients. Thus these antagonists can compound existing problems and contribute to hormonal imbalances. All of which can potentially contribute to the onset of disease and/or the progression or worsening of an already existing disorder.

Healthier Food Replacements for Traditional Denatured And/Or Devitalized Favorites

Food	Healthier Replacement
Alcohol	Dark red wine in moderation
Beer or whiskey	A glass at a special occasion

Note: Alcohol at best causes dehydration, robs the
body of essential B+Complex vitamins, and can
raise the blood pressure, and some studies have
shown how alcohol consumption can lead to
Liver disorders. The Liver is the main filtering
organ of the body.

Bleached white flour	Unbleached white flour
	Soy, Buckwheat, Millet,
	Corn, Rice, and others.

Note: Better yet, visit your local Health Food Store's
Refrigerator section, and familiarize yourself with
organic flours, nuts and grains.

Baking powder	Non-Aluminum Baking powder

Coffee	Chinese Oolong green tea, Chicory,
	or Decaf, Cocoa or unsulphured
	Molasses.

Note: Chinese green tea contains phenols, one in
particular "Catechins" have been shown in studies to
contain strong anti-viral and anti-tumor properties.

For more Food Additives information purchase: "Food Additives, Nutrients & Supplements A To Z". A title published in 1998 (Eileen Renders author) by ClearLight Publishers

Healthier Food Replacements

Hydrogenated oils   Use Extra virgin oil
(Such as Palm kernel,
Cottonseed and etc.

Saturated fat   Unsaturated fats, or good fats. Those are Omega 3, Omega 6 and are found in their highest, purest form in Organic Flax oil.

Dose: Take one tablespoonful combined with either Cottage cheese or yogurt four to five times a week.

Organic flax oil is a heart healthy supplement that can help to prevent arteriosclerosis, heart attack, plaque build up in the arteries, and is necessary for the health of the skin, hair and nails. It is also involved in the release of neurotransmitters that send and receive messages. (Always recommended for ADD and ADHD.)
Ordering information can be found in the Resource section at back of book.

Refined white sugar   Date sugar, barley malt granules, Rice malt syrup, the herb Stevia.

Synthetic estrogens   Limit intake
(Often found
in red meats)

Limit red meat consumption to about 2 to 3 times per week. Choose top quality (low fat) cuts, limit Serving sizes to approximately 3 to 4 ounces, and never fry! Bake, broil or Sauté meats.

These synthetic growth hormones are also often found in one's milk. Choose goat milk, soymilk, rice milk and/or Almond milk.

Other protein choices: Eggs, Yogurt, Soy drinks, tofu, rice and corn, rice and beans, chicken and fish.
Water ~ Have water tested, and if possible, or purchase an inexpensive water filtering system.

New and on the market is a product known as Vitamin water. Low in sugar and Sodium

Note: Consider supplementing daily requirement of Trace Minerals. A good source is granulated kelp that can be sprinkled on stews, in soups and on sandwiches.

Caution: A trace mineral is only required in minute amounts, more than ¼ teaspoon a day of kelp could trigger headaches.

Note: Prior to instituting any therapeutic nutritional supplements, it is wise to begin each day with a good multi-vitamin.

CHAPTER NINE

Specific Recommendations

Symptom	Recommendations
Anemia	Blackstrap molasses, (unsulphured), B+ Complex vitamin, especially Folic acid Sufficient protein intake.
Bloating/ Gassiness	Betaine hydrochloride (digestive-enzyme)
Cholesterol (High blood Lipid levels)	Lecithin (made from pure Soy granules only) Rice bran Complex, Red Yeast Rice

Colds & flu   Echinacea/Goldenseal, Garlic oil capsules (3-5,000 milligram capsules 3 times a day), Vitamin-C, 1,000 milligrams twice daily

Insomnia	Herbal complex containing: Skullcap, Hops, Valerian root and Passionflower. Take two capsules at bedtime.
Headache SAME-e.	Rosemary herbal tea at onset, and
	(S-adenosyl-L-methionine) 600-800 Milligrams.

**Contraindicated *in those taking MAO Inhibitors*

Constipation	Fiber: Rice bran, Bilberry, lots of water and fresh fruits

Symptoms and Recommendations continued

Diarrhea   Bilberry standardized extract is non-toxic and beneficial for either diarrhea and/or constipation. Stronger potencies for Diarrhea and less for constipation. Age and degree of severity will also help determine a beneficial dose.

Energy   EFA Essential Fatty Acids and Fat-Soluble Chlorophyll stimulates a process in the human body similar to that, which occurs in nature known as photosynthesis. The highest purest form of EFA is organic Flax oil (according to Dr. Budwig, a Nobel Prize candidate researcher). Chlorella is an herbal supplement Containing fat-soluble chlorophyll.

Immune System   Include standardization extract of the Chinese herb Astragalus root. Only the Standardization is recommended. It is 0.4% 4-Hydroxy Methody-Isoflavone 7 Sug ~ 12 drops of a liquid extract in water Twice daily, or three capsules twice daily. CO-Enzyme Q-10 ~ an antioxidant with oxygen sparing benefits; it is also an immune enhancer. 60 to 150 milligrams taken once daily is the recommendation. Shiitake mushroom extract, ascorbic acid (Natural form of vitamin-C) St. John's wort (Hypericin) a standardized extract is 300 Milligrams containing 0.3-0.5% Hypericin. Two capsules daily.

Liver Toxicity	Milk thistle (Blessed thistle) this herb contains significant amounts of Silymarin, also beneficial is organic sulfur. SAMe S-adenosylmethionine~~ this supplement has been shown to be beneficial for other disorders as well, including depression, ADD/ADHD, and fibromyaalgia. It is beneficial as well for inflammation of the joints as in Arthritis. For more information see Resources. Include high doses of vitamin-C.
Muscle weakness	Betaine as derived from the Beetroot has been shown in studies to strengthen muscles. (See Resources for Suppliers For ordering.)
Nausea	Crystallized ginger. Kuzu root~ A root starch that soothes the stomach and strengthens the intestines. Used in cooking as a thickener.
Sore Throat	SAMBUCOL ~ Elderberry syrup, Garlic oil capsules, Vitamin-C, Antiseptic mouth gargle.

Note: Doses and benefits associated with above recommendations will depend on age and seriousness of symptoms.

We strongly advise that anyone with a serious diagnosis, or taking any type of medication seek the advice of their primary care physician before taking any of the recommendations contained in this book.

We strongly advise against self-treating and caution against potential or adverse effects as a result of contraindications unknown to the individual wanting to self-treat.

****

CHAPTER TEN

Devitalized Foods and other Antagonists (To be avoided)

Over processed foods are usually those foods that have had most of their nutritional benefit removed as *live* foods are more susceptible to contamination and therefore, provide a shorter shelf life. Food additives and preservatives are used as: Colorings, anti-caking agents, anti-spoilage, for softness, texture and to inhibit mold. Synthetic compounds are often added in order to lengthen shelf life of a product.

These additives however not only do not provide the consumer with an ideal type of nutritional support that is necessary in order to support the body's daily needs, or for achieving the required optimal bodily responses for digestion, glandular support, energy needs and other responsibilities. But in fact, are antagonists that can also impose unnecessary stress upon the body's natural immune response. For example: A high sodium intake can contribute to hypertension in individuals who are sodium sensitive, or the Iodine contained in Sodium chloride (table salt) can over-stimulate the Thyroid (when consumed in excess) of a child who is hyper kinetic. Nitrates and Nitrites found in Luncheon meats, sausages, bacon, hot dogs and other cured, pickled or smoked meats can turn into a compound known as Nitrosamines. Nitrosamines are known to be potential carcinogens.

Obviously then, anyone with a known immune disorder does not need any added burden placed upon the immune system as a direct result of habitually consuming these compounds often found in devitalized foods. Phosphoric acid found in sodas can interfere with the body's ability to properly make Iron or store Calcium.

Refined white sugar by the way is a deceiving compound, for while it has a sweet taste, it is an acid. As can be noted in individuals with recurrent bouts of Candida. However, in order to arrest the symptoms of Candida, refined white sugar should be avoided like the plague. Candida is a single celled fungus known as Candida albicans, which thrives in an acidic internal environment.

ADHD Attention Deficit Hyperactive Disorder is often diagnosed in children who are hypersensitive to the chemicals often found in food additives and food preservatives. An example is the additive known as MSG, often found in Chinese foods. But, they might be just as sensitive to food colorings and food dyes as well, found in a variety of foods. A special formulation of Aluminum is often used in table Salt (Sodium chloride) and some types of flour as an additive for preventing "caking."

Hydrogenated oils are oils that have been heated to such extreme temperatures that the oil's natural molecular structure has been modified. All of the oils original benefit has been turned into a type of fat that is high on the NCI (National Cancer Institute) Suspect List of carcinogens, or free radicals that are cancer-causing agents. The very idea of a white bread that has had most of its nutrient content removed in order to lengthen shelf life is unacceptable. What nutrient content that is replaced due to the FDA (Food And Drug Administration) law is minimal, and synthetic as well. The flour that the bread, cake and rolls is made from has been processed with a type of bleach in order to whiten the bread quicker in order that it can be readily used for baking. The Baking powder often found in the Super Market also has an additive that is a derivative of Aluminum that is used for prevention of "caking." Caking is a result of any moisture due to environment, temperatures and etc.

The feed and grain that Barn yard animals usually feed on has often been sprayed with chemicals that are by some experts considered as lethal as DDT. Chemicals used as insecticides such as Heptachlor or Lindane. DDT or d *(ichloro) d (iphenyl) t (richloroethane)* is a powerful insecticide (CIC6H4) 2CHCC3 effective upon contact: law due to its damaging environmental effects restricts its use.

Beef cattle are often fed synthetic hormones that help to fatten the cows in order to bring in more dollars to the Farmers at Auction, and to get them to the Slaughterhouse more quickly. Chickens often are given potent doses of antibiotics, and all of this translates onto our dinner plate because we are only one rung up on the ladder, or link in the chain.

Just as some types of oils are higher in saturated fat, others are mono-unsaturated, poly-unsaturated, or unsaturated. Therefore, we have bad oils such as those known as hydrogenated and often found in candy bars, cookies, chips and etc. Good oils are the Essential Fatty Acids, the Linoleic and Linolenic Acids. And then there are the oils that I refer to as neutral, neither good nor bad. However we will take a closer look at some of those oils and point out those that are healthier and recommended for use in moderation.

While one might have an objection because these oils are not readily found in the local Super Markets, keep in mind that many are just as inexpensive and resources will be provided in the back of this book for purchasing healthier replacements for many of the more often used, denatured ones. Some of the benefits derived from this type of healthier food are that they actually help to lower blood lipid levels, satisfy hunger, help to prevent unwanted weight gain, and thereby help to prevent heart disease and/or type-2 diabetes.

These benefits by the way are achievable, as well as many other benefits. All without compromising the liver, the body's natural detoxifying organ. More information on Food Additives can be found in a title I authored back in 1999 for CLEAR LIGHT PUBLISHERS appropriately titled: Food Additives, Nutrients And Supplements A To Z, A Shopper's Guide. This book alphabetizes five chapters and is a good reference source for familiarizing oneself with the good and the bad food additives. It sells for $14.95. Or log onto www.NaturalHealingDr.com.

Understanding how these denatured foods can become antagonistic to optimum health of the human body, and how they not only contribute to the onset of various common disorders (or worsen the severity of them), but also will provide understanding on how these chemicals can also inhibit the body's own natural healing response.

So let us now move on and provide you with a partial list of foods that are best avoided, and include suggestions for healthier replacement foods. The healthier food suggestions it should be mentioned however, not only eliminate the *antagonistic factor,* but also provide the missing element often necessary for helping the body to heal. Many of the following foods listed here can be therapeutic when taken in the proper concentrated dose as recommended by your Health Care practitioner in order to address symptoms associated with specific common disorders.

Because various herbs and or concentrated supplements are employed therapeutically and often temporarily in order to effect a desired change, it is advised that one seeks proper advisement. For in some instances, these very supplements could trigger a nutritional imbalance when dose and/or a skilled practitioner is not supervising duration. Therefore, it is strongly advised that readers do not decide to self-treat.

A Naturopath, Nutritionist or Doctor of Naturopathy is a good place to seek advice.

Foods that are on the "Suspect List of carcinogens"

Caffeine:
Decaffeinated
Coffee
Fat
Food Additives
Hair dye
Herbicides
Hydrogenated oils: Pam kernel, cottonseed oil, mostly found in junk foods such as candy bars, cookies, cakes, pies and etc.
Indoor Air quality
Involuntary Smoking
Microwave oven
Mouthwash
Nitrate
Nitrite
Nitrosamines
Nuclear Power Plant
Radon
Saccharin ~ As well as most sugar substitutes
Smoking
Ultraviolet Radiation

Note: The above is a partial list and other information can be obtained through the National Institutes of Health or The American Cancer Society.

A List of Denatured and Devitalized Foods that can antagonize and/or contribute to symptoms associated with many disorders:

Alcohol
Caffeine
Cigarettes
Fried foods ~ (When consumed in excess, or when fried using hydrogenated oils.)
Hydrogenated oils ~ Oils that have been treated in such high temperatures that their molecular structure has been changed. Thereby turning harmless oils into dangerous free radicals.
Luncheon meats: Bologna, Salami, & etc. are high in **Nitrates and Nitrites** which when consumed begin to transform into Nitrosamines in the intestines, and they are known carcinogens.

Note: Vitamin-C helps to eliminate, or render Nitrosamines harmless, especially when taken at time such foods are eaten.

Overly processed foods: Usually found in boxes, bags and/or cans. Or they could simply be prepared foods with cream sauces with high saturated fat and/or Sodium content. Make it a perpetual habit to read all ingredient labels.
Prepared foods: Usually devoid of nutrients, but Saturated with Sodium chloride (table Salt), saturated fats and food colorings and other additives.
Refined white flour: And all products made from it: Breads, pies, cakes, rolls, and cookies. Refined white flour has bleaching agents, an Aluminum source for preventing caking, and is devoid of nutrients.

Refined white sugar: Avoid refined white sugar, as well as all products made from refined white sugar. This includes bakery products, soda, candy, and other denatured foods.

Note: Refined white sugar is an overly processed sugar that is acidic and can be detrimental in contributing to an overly acidic internal environment. An overly acidic internal environment can be conducive to the type of environment that precludes many types of problems: Candida, ulcers or even cancer.

Excess consumption can deplete the body's ability to retain and/or store adequate amounts of the essential B+Complex vitamins.

Smoked Meats: Sausages, hams, hot dogs, bacon and hams.

ELEVEN

Healthier Food Replacements for Devitalized Foods & other Antagonists

Denatured food	Healthier replacement
White flour and all products made from white made from white flour.	Stone ground, whole grains, such as Millet, Soy, and Corn Buckwheat, Garbanzo bean flour and more. Keep Refrigerated, as these flours are alive.
Caffeine drinks	Chickory, Chinese Oolong Green tea, and concentrated fruit Juices without added sugar.
Cooking oils	Preferably Extra virgin olive oil. Almond oil, walnut oil.
Fried foods	Sautee' in low Sodium chicken bullion, or light cooking wine.
Luncheon meats	Egg salad, homemade soups, Salads, dinner Leftovers, yogurt or Soy Protein drinks.
Milk	Organic low-fat milk, Soymilk, Goat's milk, Rice or Almond milk.

Note: Rice bran oil has been shown to lower LDL blood lipid levels about 30% without causing any toxicity to the Liver, as well as other benefits.

Denatured food	Healthier replacement
Processed foods	Fresh fruits and vegetables in Season, organic or pre-cleaned.

Denatured or highly processed foods are usually found in a box, a bag or a can.

Note: Products that remove 99% of pesticide residues Are often found in your Supermarket's produce section, or at a Health Food store. Proctor Gamble known as "Fit" makes one such product.

Saturated fat	Avoid or limit
Red meat	A perfect food source containing all of the essential Amino acids that constitute a perfect protein. Essential Amino acids are necessary in order to insure sufficient Protein intake is adequate, and for the prevention of anemia.

Note: Red meat may be a double edge sword however, because while it is considered by many authorities to be a perfect protein, it is also usually high in saturated fat.

Other healthy forms of protein include

Eggs	Soy	Cheese
Chicken	Fish	Rice and corn
Chickpeas	Yogurt	Rice and beans
Protein drinks		Egg whites
Egg substitute		Tofu

Note: Although red meat is a perfect protein, it need not be eaten daily in order to supply the body's need for protein. To reduce the amount of fat in red meat, select top cuts; trim fat and broil rather than fry. A portion would be about 3 to 4 ounces, or not more than the size of one's fist. Often high in saturated fat, red meat often contains synthetic growth hormones used to fatten the cattle in order to command higher prices at the Market.

Sodas: Instead opt for diluted or double diluted concentrated fruit juices, Chinese Oolong Green tea with a dash of your Favorite flavoring extract such as Mint, Vanilla or Lemon. This can also be a great opportunity for fruit intake when added to your teas or in a Protein shake.

****

CHAPTER TWELVE

Prescribed Drugs used in the Treatment of HIV/AIDS

AZT also known as Zidovudine is the first anti-HIV drug to be used in the treatment of HIV/AIDS. Burroughs Wellcome manufactures this drug through a brand name Retrovir. Because this drug is metabolized by the body's Liver and eliminated through the kidneys, it is to be prescribed with caution for patients with Liver and/or kidney disorders.

Side effects include: Headache, hypertension, anxiety, muscle weakness, diarrhea and for some, insomnia.

Note: Because AZT is eliminated via the kidneys; the simultaneous use of other toxic drugs can potentially increase the risk of serious side effects. Some of these toxic drugs include Clarithromycin, amphotericin B, dapsone, vincristine, flucytosine, vinblastine and Adriamycin or interferon. These drugs are often used to treat infection, and may therefore, often be used by patient's with HIV. Some of these drugs increase the AZT levels in the blood while others decrease its availability, and dosage of AZT will require adjustment.

While AZT has been shown to moderately raise CD4+ counts and reduce the number of opportunistic infections and other symptoms of HIV infection in individuals with CD4+ counts lower than 200, and in people with higher counts who may be symptomatic, studies suggest however, over an extended period of time, AZT used alone loses its effectiveness. Possibly as with various other medications, the body builds up a tolerance to the drug.

DDC ~ Dideoxycytidine or zalcitabine is sold under the drug name of Hivid, Manufacturer: Rachel. This drug has been used for the treatment of HIV in adults with advanced HIV disease who are intolerant to AZT, or have disease progression while receiving AZT. It has also been used in conjunction with AZT for the treatment of advanced HIV disease.

This drug also has its own set of side effects, and is not a cure for HIV. In fact, HIV progression or opportunistic infections while taking DDC may continue to progress.

Side effects can be serious or miniscule. On the serious side, Peripheral neuropathy is a potential possibility, and is a nerve damage that includes: Numbness, tingling and/or sharp burning in the feet legs and hands. Patients experiencing any of these symptoms while on this medication should contact their physician immediately. Of the Volunteers taking DDC in a study, 25 to 35% experienced neuropathy. If caught early, these symptoms are said to be temporary or reversible. Pancreatic disease is another serious potential side effect of taking DDC, however those affected are reported to be slightly higher than 1%.

This drug will have negative side effects when taken in conjunction with amino glycoside antibiotics, amphotericin B, anticancer drugs, dapsone, riboflavin and many other drugs.

DDL or Didanosine: dideoxyinosine.

This drug falls under the drug name of Videx and is manufactured by Bristol/Myers Squibb Oncology. It has been used in the treatment of advanced HIV disease in adults. It is also approved in lower dose forms for children with HIV. With its own set of side effects, it is often more tolerable to patients whose constitution cannot tolerate the side effects of AZT. Again this drug may not be well tolerated, especially by individuals with a hypersensitivity to aspartame, as it is contained in this drug. DDL can cause severe disease of the pancreas (pancreatitis) and should be used with caution as this can and has been fatal in some cases.

DDL is also associated with peripheral neuropathy, a nerve disorder that is associated with numbness. Individuals with liver or kidney problems are indeed at an increased risk for developing neuropathy as a result of taking DDL.

Diarrhea is often a common side effect of this drug, and can often be severe. Other side effects that occur in more than 5% of drug users are: Skin rashes, abdominal pain, nausea/vomiting, chills and fever, infection and liver failure.

D4T ~ Stavudine, didehydro-eoxythymidine.

The brand name is Zerit, and the Manufacturer is Bristol-Myers Squibb Oncology. It is used for individuals with advanced HIV disease who may be intolerant of, or who have not found beneficial treatment through the use of other antiretroviral therapies. (And as with most other drugs, D4T is metabolized in the liver, and should therefore, not be used by patients with any liver disorders.

Side effects ~ the more serious side effects include; peripheral neuropathy, and with this particular drug, more than 21% experienced this side effect when using D4T.

Similar to AZT, D4T also appears to interfere with the bone marrow's ability to produce specific white blood cells, namely neutrophils. This side effect is said to rarely occur. Other side effects include: (from Clinical trials) dry skin, fungal infections and an elevation in liver enzymes indicating possible liver toxicity.

FAMCICLOVIR ~ Famvir, Manufactured by SmithKline Beecham.

This Class of drug is used and approved for the treatment of acute herpes zoster (shingles) caused by varicella-zoster virus VZV. This drug is approved only for use in the treatment of herpes zoster. Side effects are said to be few, including headache, fatigue, and nausea.

FOSCARNET ~ Sold under the drug name of Foscavir, it is Manufactured by Astra.

The FDA has approved foscarnet in the treatment of cytomegalovirus (CMV) retinitis of people with AIDS. While it has not been approved to treat infections caused by herpes simplex virus (HSV), and varicella-zoster virus (VZV), it is used when the drug of choice acyclovir, is not effective or cannot be tolerated by the patient. While the drug does not stop the progression of the disease (retinitis), it can often delay its progression.

Cautions: Large doses can increase the toxicity of the drug and of course, many patients may be hypersensitive to this class of drugs.

Side effects most prevalent to individuals taking this drug include some level of kidney toxicity. At least one third of volunteers (individuals with AIDS) developed serious kidney problems when taking this drug. Foscarnet is also known to lead to changes in minerals and electrolytes in the blood, which have triggered seizures. Electrolyte imbalance is a serious and sometimes fatal side effect of foscarnet.

Warning signs include: Burning an/or prickling sensations, numbness in the mouth and seizures. Other side effects include: Confusion, coughing, abdominal pain, depression, anxiety, nausea, diarrhea, rash, vomiting, dizziness, increased sweating and/or difficulty breathing.

**GANCICLOVIR ~ DHPG, Brand name is
Cytovene and it is Manufactured by Syntex.**

Ganciclovir has been approved for treatment of
cytomegalovirus (CMV) retinitis in people with a
compromised immune system. This drug is also used
for the prevention of wider range of CMV diseases in
patients receiving organ or tissue transplants. While
Ganciclovir is not a cure for CMV retinitis, it has been
shown to interfere with the multiplication of CMV,
thus slowing down the disease and/or further
destruction of the retina.

Great Caution is warned for individuals with HIV
who take this drug as it has been found to interfere
with the bone marrow's ability to manufacture
neutrophils and platelets. And a loss of decrease of
neutrophils and platelets will significantly raise one's
risk for developing an infection. For certain, this may
be the greatest risk in using Cytovene.

3TC ~ Lamivudine ~ An Antiviral Experimental drug
for HIV, it is also being studied for the treatment of
Hepatitis B. There is not much information available
regarding drug interactions, nor how this drug will
react in the elderly or in children.

Side effects of 3TC are nausea in 15 to 25% (as
noted in Clinical trials), headache. High doses have
caused serious deficiencies in neutrophils (white blood
cells), which remarkably raise the risk for infection.

OTHER HIV TREATMENT DRUGS

Human Growth Hormone and Steroids have been used in HIV patients as an Anti-wasting measure when 10% or more of lean body mass is lost, especially when CD4+ counts plummet to, or below 100.

It is well documented that anabolic steroids are associated with a type of water retention that raises the blood volume, which in turn can often cause weight gain and hypertension. Steroids have been linked to gastrointestinal problems, including ulcers and/or internal bleeding.

Growth Hormone treatment is still under study, or the final word with regard to its exact benefit verses its potential harm is still being evaluated. See more information on Growth Hormone in this chapter under "Growth Hormone."

DRONABINOL ~ Delta-9-THC is listed under the brand name of Marinol, and is manufactured by Roxane.

Dronabinol is utilized to address weight loss in the HIV patient due to loss of appetite. It also has been a method of treatment for nausea resulting from chemotherapy resulting from cancer. This drug is a central nervous system depressant and can compromise one's ability to operate any machinery, including an automobile. It should not be used in conjunction with alcohol, or any other barbiturate such as Valium. Also, this drug has an effect on the nervous system and can potentiate mania, depression or schizophrenia.

Because this drug may cause low blood pressure (or rapid heartbeat or fainting), in individuals with a history of heart disease, it should be used with extreme caution under strict supervision.

Side effects for this drug include: Giddiness, confusion, drowsiness, and/or dizziness. These symptoms may be dose related, and are said to cease when the drug is discontinued.

HUMAN GROWTH HORMONE (RHGH) ~ HGH, r-HGH, somatrem, somatropin. Known as Humatrope by Lily, Protropin by Genentech, and Serostim by Seronol.

This drug has been used in treating children who have been diagnosed with a growth hormone deficiency, and do not grow normally.

Because this is a synthetic hormone it has been linked to stimulating growth of any active tumors, especially in people who have cancer that is not under control.

Side effects ~ rHGH has been thought to lead to the development of antibodies to growth hormones found naturally in the body. Clinical trials in using rHGH in the treatment of wasting diseases have these side effects: Swelling, joint stiffness, raised tryglyceride blood levels, and nausea. Many of these side effects were reversed when the dose was adjusted.

MEGESTROL ~ Megace, by Bristol-Myers Squibb Oncology. This drug is a synthetic hormone-appetite stimulant. Weight loss in HIV patients can be common as it can be triggered by opportunistic infections that become antagonistic to the natural ability of the intestines to fully absorb nutrients ingested.

Cautions indicate that Megestrol is only to be Used <u>after</u> infections, or other poor nutrition possibilities have first been addressed. This drug should not be used to prevent weight loss, as there is no evidence proving that the drug is effective in accomplishing this.

Volunteers in clinical trials reported diarrhea, rash, gas, impotence, insomnia, nausea and high blood pressure. However it is noted that individuals receiving a placebo reported the same side effects as often as those who had been taking the actual drug. More rarely, Megestrol caused blood clotting in the legs. Other side effects include: Decreased testosterone levels, and breast enlargement in men.

Final Note:

There are literally dozens of other drugs used in the treatment of HIV, some of those drugs are used to treat other accompanying conditions separate from HIV, and others of these drugs are used ironically to treat the side effects associated with the primary treatment drugs. Could it be that one day there will be new drugs to treat the side effects that are resulting from the drugs used to treat the side effects resulting from the primary drugs used in the treatment of HIV?

The bottom line is this: By the time an individual reaches the age of say 40 to 45 years of age, the main filtering organ of the human body (one's Liver) is now only capable of functioning at perhaps 45 to 55% capacity as it once did at the age of 18 to 20 years of age.

It is clear that each synthetic drug used in the treatment of HIV/AIDS has proven itself to be a potent drug with a proven toxicity! When these drugs begin to accumulate in the body's liver, and are not being adequately eliminated, the result is what I often refer to as an *accumulative effect!*

When the liver is toxic it is understandable that this toxicity will further weaken the immune system. Considering how HIV/AIDS is a disease of the immune system, it appears that the traditional treatment used thus far in the treatment of HIV leaves a lot to be desired!

Once again, allow me to call your attention to a fact that was mentioned earlier on in this book, but one that will be proven to be one of the most important facts you will read in this book, a fact that is therefore, worth repeating.

Sunday, February 4, 2001 (more than 2 ½ years ago), THE HERALD-TRIBUNE, a Newspaper of New Jersey printed an article it had taken from The New York Times News Service. We will provide that article for your review, word for word, in its entirety.

"CHICAGO News" - Altering a long held policy, Federal health officials now recommend that treatment for the AIDS virus be delayed as long as possible for people without symptoms because of increased concerns over toxic effects of the drug therapies being used at that time!

The new guidelines, written by a federal panel and due to be announced Monday, represent a major philosophical shift in treating HIV, the AIDS virus.

Instead of the *Hit early, hit hard* approach in effect since 1996, the new approach calls for waiting until the Immune system shows serious signs of weakening or HIV levels in the blood far exceed those for which treatment is recommended.

The panel, convened by the Department of Health and Human Services and the Henry J. Kaiser Family Foundation, still recommends therapy for anyone who develops symptoms of AIDS.

Therapy should also be given to people whose blood tests show they have been infected for less than six months, in the belief that early treatment might strengthen the immune system's ability to fight the virus, the panel says.

Such guidelines have no force of law. Wide-scale application would mean that some infected people might defer costly therapy for up to three years and ultimately decrease the risk of toxicities, said Dr. Anthony S. Fauci, director of the National Institute of Allergy and Infectious Diseases.

The aggressive approach to treating HIV was adopted shortly after protease inhibitor drugs were marketed and then combined with older drugs in 1996.

These drug cocktails, which suppress the amount of HIV in the blood beyond levels that tests could detect, led to substantial responses, with many AIDS patients getting off their deathbeds or going back to work.

Yet many experts advocated early treatment for healthy infected people to prevent damage to the immune system.

A few Virologists raised hopes that in a short time the drugs might eliminate HIV from the body, thus achieving a cure and obviating any drug therapy. However studies show that the drug cocktails do not cure HIV, and when infected people stop therapy, the virus rebounds, making lifetime therapy necessary.

More recently, concern has grown over nerve damage, weakened bones, unusual accumulations of fat in the neck and abdomen, diabetes and a number of other serious side effects of therapy.

Many people have developed dangerously high levels of cholesterol and other lipids in the blood, raising concern that HIV-infected people might face yet another epidemic--heart disease.

The pendulum has swung from when few therapies were available and most people died from AIDS to a time when drug cocktails are effective but creating complications.

"We are adopting a significantly more conservative recommendation profile, one that allows the virus to remain in the body longer in return for sparing the patient the drug toxicities" said Fauci, who is co-chairman of the panel as stated in an interview.

****

CHAPTER THIRTEEN

Tracking Bernie's Progress (and problems)

The first time I met Bernie, I must admit that I did have some apprehension. Bernie is not his real name as all names have been changed in order to protect privacy.)

Although Renders Wellness has an office Suite that is attached to our home and situated on four pristine acres, at the time Renders Wellness was sub-contracted through The Atlantic City Medical Center's HIV Consortium, our new office was under construction and I was working out of a Trailer in the backyard. Quiet and serene it is, yet somewhat solitary in that woods surround it. There is a small church to the left and the property to the right is about a quarter mile away.

Meanwhile just before construction was about to begin for our new home and office, Renders Wellness' shingle hung on a Trailer. Working diligently, I set out preparing audio tapes for Guided Imagery sessions, and set up new file cabinets and preparing duplicate forms that would be used for each new client. Renders Wellness would be responsible for Guided Imagery sessions, Nutritional support and Herbal recommendations.

Putting together a protocol would be no easy task. There would be general recommendations, as well as specific recommendations.

Our involvement would be to support the HIV/AIDS population of two (2) counties in New Jersey, Atlantic County and Cape May County.

As busy as I was in those first days, I was also aware of being very much alone on the grounds, and sensed a vulnerability that was not familiar to me.

My first appointment was with a client who was not only of the opposite sex, and of a different race, but was from a different community and of course, HIV. Not sure exactly what to expect I pondered, would he be angry? Was he high on drugs? As the hour drew near, I felt somewhat comforted in knowing that only drug free applicants were qualified to participate and be accepted into the program.

The irony of it all is that this is the one individual who later turned out to be the only HIV patient who remained in the Renders Wellness program long after Renders Wellness left The Atlantic City Medical Center's HIV Consortium. Today, after eight years in our care, however, I can tell you that Bernie and I have shared much about life, family and spirituality. In fact, I later confessed to Bernie the anxiety I had felt that first day long ago when first we met. We were then able to share a laugh about it. Bernie was open and shared a lot about himself with me, and I wanted to seal that trust by sharing a part of myself too! Bernie like myself had a lot of faith and trust in God.

Bernie completed all of the necessary paperwork back in 1995 or 1996, including bringing with him copies of recent lab work that he had done in the weeks preceding our first Consultation. It was at that time, Bernie revealed to me how he had been on AZT for nearly a year, but had been constantly plagued with symptoms such as diarrhea, muscle weakness, headache, insomnia, nausea and loss of energy. He went on to share with me that although he had been diagnosed with the HIV virus nearly five years previous to our meeting, he had only taken the drug for one year. He openly discussed with me that he had recently decided that he would rather die than live a life that left him feeling incapacitated, or without hope.

Bernie also confessed that when Renders Wellness was added to the Program as Adjuvant services, he had made a quiet decision that he intended to carry out. This decision was to go off of drug therapy entirely!

Knowing that any influence on my part was illegal, and far from any thoughts of my own, Bernie's words came as somewhat of a shock to me (especially since our program and protocol was just getting off the ground). I felt it was my responsibility to insist that he remain on drug therapy. Bernie however, was just as insistent that he did not wish to remain on drug therapy, and made reference to the fact that it was his right to make the final decision. And there was nothing left for me to do at that point, other than to respect his rights and wishes, as well as his privacy.

However, before Bernie left that day, I asked him to at least relay the same information to his medical physician as he had just shared with me, and the discussion was over. Bernie's drug therapy was between The Infectious Disease Center and Bernie. My responsibility on the other hand, was to make Bernie aware of how stress could weaken the immune system, and to teach him a method of Guided Imagery, nutritionally support him, and assist him in boosting his immune system, as well as educate him with regard to detoxification of the liver.

His understanding regarding how antagonists could interfere with the internal balance, (homeostasis) or action and reactions soon became his motivation for adopting healthier eating habits, managing his stress, and continuing to regard his daily recommendations (which were many) of supplements as his life-line. Bernie didn't smoke cigarettes and didn't drink alcohol.

And now he was learning that he must also avoid refined white sugar and limit coffee intake to one cup a day. There was one problem however, that Bernie needed to correct. That was his occasional use of marijuana. We explained to Bernie how one "joint" of marijuana was equal to one pack of cigarettes with regard to its negative effect upon the lungs. Then we told him this drug is often laced with other chemicals in order to produce the temporary high that was meant not only to entice the user, but also to keep them dependent upon the drug. It was explained to Bernie how these toxins could accumulate within the liver and lead to a further weakening of the immune system. All of which Bernie was reminded, could set the stage for vulnerability making him much more susceptible to other serious problems. And of course, these actions are counter-productive!

Before leaving our office, Bernie was given a whole list of nutrients and herbal supplements he needed to purchase and was reminded that he needed to take them every day without fail if he truly expected to reap the full benefit.

After Bernie left my office, I began to scope out all of his Lab results he had brought with him while paying special attention to the viral load, and T-4 counts. These would be the figures (present and future) that would tell the story of how well Bernie was managing his disease, or if any progression could be noted.

Another appointment had been scheduled for the month ahead, and after his next blood work was to be done. In that way, we could compare progress and make adjustments and/or corrections to his recommendations.

Bernie remained faithful to the recommendations made to him that day, and it was his intention to avoid taking the potent AZT drug to which he had many aversions.

In those first few months into his program, Bernie appeared to be holding his own. By that I mean that his viral load and T-Counts appeared to be stabilized. But over the Holidays of that first Christmas as Bernie followed the program, we received a telephone call from him stating that he had swollen glands and a sore throat. From the tone of his voice it was evident that Bernie also was dealing with a great deal of fear.

Would he be able to avoid a serious illness? Might he now become hospitalized because he had decided not to continue taking the medications his medical physician at the Infectious Disease Center had prescribed for him?

Although I could hear the fear in his voice, at that time I was not yet aware of the reason for such fear. And it was some time before Bernie confirmed for me that he had indeed, stopped all prescribed medications. Later, I learned from Bernie how he did not want anyone to know that he was drug free because he feared he would be kicked out of the program. That for Bernie, would mean no more free supplements and free blood work.

And of course, he had concern that should he become really ill or be hospitalized, he would have to confess to his primary care physician that he had not been faithful to taking his prescribed medications. While his medications were also of no charge to him, apparently there was no one tracking whether these prescriptions were being filled or not. Therefore, no one could say who was, or who was not taking his/her medications.

All things considered, I suggested to Bernie that perhaps he ought to call his medical doctor and obtain an antibiotic prescription. "No" Bernie replied, "I can't do that!" And I asked him why not. "Because, the doctor doesn't want us to keep taking antibiotics because of the side effects, and because should there come a time when we really need to depend on them, they won't have as great a benefit to offer due to our tolerance level being affected!"

Since it was the weekend, I instructed him to double up on all of his natural recommendations, and remain at home and off of his feet. He was instructed that if he felt no better in a day or two, to see his medical physician.

Two days later, Bernie telephoned me all excited, saying: "Eileen, the potent garlic oil capsules and the double dosing of my Astragalus Root Extract worked, my swollen glands and sore throat are gone!"

Well if Bernie had not been a believer before, he was now a follower! With the next couple of Lab results, it became obvious that Bernie's viral load had been reduced to nearly half of what it had been when first he entered into the program at Renders Wellness. While Bernie's HIV was always evident in his Lab results, his T-4 cells had become stronger. In fact, at times it really just bordered on the low end of what was considered normal.

While it was still early in the game, it looked as though his new recommendations were working for him. More importantly, Bernie felt better than he had in years. True, he had to avoid refined white sugar, white bread, alcohol, cigarettes and hydrogenated oils, but he was making progress in learning how to obtain some of the tastes and flavors he enjoyed, without resorting to those that might contribute to his disease.

With Bernie's faith in God and his trust in his fellow man, he all work for the glory of God. Bernie is always ready to discuss the topic of faith. His determination and ability to follow direction in remaining constant to his program and health goals is probably what sets him apart from many others. The power of faith and trust in God cannot be trivialized. Each time we reviewed Bernie's blood work that came to us from the Laboratory seemed to reaffirm Bernie's belief that healing requires faith.

In just six month's his viral load had gone down from 135,000 milligrams per deciliter to 36,000 mpd. His T-Counts (T-4 & etc) had risen to a point where it just hovered below the bottom of the scale that is referred to as "normal." For Bernie it appeared that the program was working, and he was making it work! Renders Wellness for the most part was the educator and motivator, but it was Bernie who did all the work.

Bernie's progress was followed from 1995 and is still being followed today in 2004. A man who was diagnosed HIV In 1989, Bernie is a man who works, drives a car, helps others and at forty-eight years of age weighs in at 185 pounds. And Bernie has not been hospitalized in over eight years!

At the time of our first meeting, Bernie had been plagued with chronic diarrhea, constipation, insomnia, and muscle weakness and did his attending physician at the Infectious Disease Center prescribe taking AZT.

While The Infectious Disease Center has since adopted other ways of mapping the disease, including the use of markers that are now being adopted with regard to the prescribing of various medications (including potencies of same), at that time medications were being prescribed across the board, regardless of staging. However, at some point in time and after several years of following the Renders Wellness protocol, Bernie openly admits that he had stopped taking all medication shortly after coming into the program.

We were obliged not to share that information with his primary care physician and to protect his right to privacy, but did urge him to share that information with his primary care physician at the Infectious Disease Center.

While on AZT in 1995, we noted that Bernie's Mature T (CD3) was at 78 (the norm being between 62-87. Absolute CD3+ was 1170 while norm was 630-3170.

His Helper (CD-4+) was 33 that were good as norm was between 32-62. His Absolute CD4+ was at 495, and considered on the low end as norm was 400-1770. CD8 was excellent, on the high end and the Absolute CD8 was at the half way marker. Everything was looking pretty good, however Bernie felt as though he was truly dying!

Therefore, it is important to note that the quality of life is what makes life worth living. Living a happy and productive life! That is exactly however, what Bernie had reportedly been missing in his life previously. Tracking Bernie we found him to remain on the low end of normal ranges for most chemistry results, but he on the other hand, reported a relief of symptoms such as diarrhea, nausea, insomnia, headache, and muscle ache and had begun working part time. That was a step forward!

Bernie also had a problem with his red blood cells and it was difficult to treat his anemia, as he did not always respond ideally to his prescribed iron supplement. In fact, as far as anemia was concerned, his condition (results) often vacillated between anemia and "borderline."

In 1998, Bernie continued to show favorable T-Counts and lowered viral loads, unless of course, he was fighting a cold or sinus infection that would temporarily be evident in his Lab results. During those times, we doubled up on our recommendation doses, and advised Bernie to remain at home and at rest.

Along with Bernie's anemia problem, there was also a diagnosed hypertension problem. Once again, Bernie objected to taking the medication prescribed for lowering his blood pressure. However, we were able to successfully convince him of the increased risk he was taking for heart attack and/or stroke in not taking his scripts.

In 1999 Bernie's viral load went up to about 71,000 milligrams per deciliter which was well above the 18 to 36,000 milligrams per deciliter that we had been seeing, but was still well below the 136,000 milligrams per deciliter we had seen earlier on back in 1995 and 1996.

Throughout 1999 we saw some better Absolute CD4 results, and the viral load readings fluctuated within acceptable ranges; his attending medical physician was continuing to treat Bernie for his high blood pressure.

His anemia however, never seemed to be resolved completely. Nor was it resolved for any extended period of time. At that time, we supported his anemia through recommendation of Black Strap molasses (unsulphured). It is often an ideal recommendation for individuals who are unable to tolerate the B+ complex vitamin. Black Strap molasses is high in iron and many of the B Complex vitamins, including several essential minerals.

In order to provide some support for his hypertension, we recommended Calcium/Magnesium and the essential enzyme know as CO-Enzyme Q-10. We also guided him toward foods that contained a fair supply of Calcium and Magnesium, as we did not want him to rely totally on supplements, but to encourage him to make healthier lifestyle changes that would become permanent changes in his life.

Dark green vegetables, we pointed out were ideal, as they also contained Folic Acid which was essential f or making healthy red blood cells, as well as helping to insure the absorption of the Calcium he needed.

In 2001 Bernie was given the HIV-1 GENOTYPING FOR DRUG RESISTANCE TO PRI. This is a Test that is done to discover whether or not an individual shows resistance to the drug, and if so the 3rd generation of Copies that has been detected. While this Test was not cleared or approved by U.S. Food and Drug Administration, the FDA had determined that such clearance or approval was not necessary.

Because Bernie had not been on any drug therapy, the Results of this Test certainly could not be conclusive regarding the 3RD generation of copies with relationship to drug therapy.

However, it should be said that these results are on average showing a one to threefold increase of higher results as from the previous essays. In other words, a less than threefold increase in HIV-1 RNA level most likely represented a new, re-standardized set point for the patient. A result that increased in excess of threefold could represent a real increase in viral load. Retesting within one to four weeks to verify the new baseline should be considered. Bernie came in slightly more than two-fold. Showing therefore, that he was still "holding his own."

In May of 2001 Bernie's viral load doubled from 32,400 milligrams per deciliter to 62,900 milligrams per deciliter. Yet his Lymphocytes and CD4's were actually a bit better than the last Testing. In talking with Bernie during one of our regular office visits we discovered that he had been pushing himself too hard at work, working more hours than usual due to a need for more money. His automobile needed repair and he was in a very negative personal relationship. We talked about all of that, and of course his nutritional intake, as well as his consistent taking of his supplements (concentrated nutrients and herbs) on a regular daily basis. He assured me that nothing had changed in that department, as he continued to remain faithful to his regime.

Therefore, we determined that he needed to make the necessary changes in his personal life that would lessen or eliminate the stress he was feeling. Stress alone can often be the culprit in causing a loss of nutrients, sleep, energy and contribute to the weakening of the immune response!

Once Bernie saw in black and white through Lab. reports how the stress affected his health, he was better able to draw limits and boundaries within relationships that allowed him to proceed confidently, and without guilt. He was motivated to take control of his life.

Another problem plaguing Bernie was his allergies. We recommended a Bioflavonoid complex to be taken with his Ascorbic Acid (natural vitamin –C), and often reminded him of the importance of taking his daily Essential Fatty Acid supplement. We also advised him to regularly use a Saline solution spray whenever he experienced stuffiness or nasal drip in order to prevent a recurrent Sinus infection. Too, he would take a high potency Garlic capsule (5,000 milligrams) several times a day. Garlic's organic sulfur content also helped to excrete toxins from the body.

91

In October 2001 Bernie's Serology-Immunology collection results looked like this:

		Normal range
Mature T (CD3)		57-85
Absolute CD 3+1155		840-3060
Helper CD 4+30		30-61
Absolute CD4+474		490-1740
Suppress (CD8) 40		12-42
Absolute CD8+644		180-1170
Helper Suppressor 0.75		0.86-5.00
Absol Lymph CT 1590		850-1000

Bernie's HIV-1 RNA quantitation (new way of Testing) was 7.157 copies x 10/ml. In January 2002 Bernie's Serology Immunology collection results looked like the following.

	Normal range
Mature (CD3) 74	57-85
ABSOLUTE CD3 +1059	840-3060
Helper (CD4+) 30	30-61
Absolute CD4+435	490-1740
SUPPRESS (CD8+) 44	12-42
Absolute (CD8+) 628	180-1170
Helper Suppressor 0.68	0.86-5.00
Absol Lymph CT 1440	850-3900

HIV-1 RNA quantitation is 9.296 copies x 10/ml

While Bernie's noticeable changes are important they are not severe, and as mentioned earlier are prone to fluctuate with each new result. Sometimes a bit higher, and then a slight fall may again be noted.

Another way of looking at it would be to review his Viral load ~ Treatment Regimen Flow Sheet.

Date	Viral load	CD-4	Treatment
11/13/96	49,130	284	AZT
02/19/97	211,571	362	AZT + Natural Protocol
09/12/97	115,516	312	Natural only
01/30/98	37,812	492	Natural Supplements Plus herbs

Note: It is important to note here that while Bernie was using only natural concentrated supplements, diet and herbs to manage his HIV viral load, he still had not yet relayed as much to the Infectious Disease Center, or his primary care physician. Bernie had fears that he would be eliminated from the program were he to make known this information to the Consortium.

Above all, Bernie feared losing the benefits that accompanied involvement in the program. Benefits such as the regular blood screenings he was getting in order to monitor his level of disease, as well as the supplements that he remained faithful to.

Viral Load – Treatment Regimen Flow Sheet Cont'd

Date	Viral load	CD-4 Count	Treatment
10/02/98	18,800	462	AZT

93

Without taking the two prescribed drugs

12/30/98	42,479	487	Natural
02/11/99	71,568	365	same

Note: It was about the same time, or perhaps a bit earlier when Bernie began to hint to his attending medical physician that he did not believe in the drugs and furthermore, was not at all consistent in taking them.

As relayed to us by Bernie, his physician expressed to him how irresponsible a decision this was, and how it could affect him seriously if he did not reconsider.

Date	Viral load	CD-4	Treatment
5/27/99	18,036	462	Same (Natural)
12/01/99	87,189	352	Ditto

It was again at this time that Bernie relayed to his physician that he was indeed not taking any medication, felt wonderful and had no intention of going back on medication. Bernie questioned his physician now (mustering up all the nerve he could manage) about *why* he wanted him on toxic drugs that came with serious side effects when he was not only getting good results, but also feeling excellent. The answers Bernie got did not convince him to reverse his decision regarding the drugs.

Date	Viral load	CD-4 Count	Treatment
4/19/00	85,000	313	AZT
7/24/00	46,200	467	Ditto
10/16/01	7,157	474	none prescribed

In Bernie's words, no medications were prescribed at this time. It is not difficult to see why Bernie continued to believe that he made the right decision for himself when he decided to stop all potent drugs for the treatment of his HIV.

Perhaps it is no coincidence that there is a definite parallel between our findings and what the Federal Health panel now suggests with regard to treating HIV.
As mentioned earlier on (Chapter 12, pages 80/81)) we included a verbatim article that was printed in the Herald-Tribune (N.J. Newspaper) in 2001, as they quoted what had been printed in the New York Times News Service. The New York Times News Service printed an article that came out of Chicago and told how the Federal Health Panel early on in 1996 had set up guidelines for treating HIV/AIDS with potent medications saying: "Hit early, hit hard!"

However in 2001 and after reviewing the results of their original recommendations and the effects of them, they wanted to change their earlier guidelines. The aggressive treatments with potent toxic drugs it appears had brought about much concern as many of these individuals taking these drug cocktails had virus rebounds, nerve damage, weakened bones, unusual fat accumulations in the neck and abdomen, diabetes, high cholesterol (some leading to heart disease) and other potential problems.

So the pendulum had swung, and they realized that from a time when there were few therapies available and people died from AIDS, to a time when drug cocktails were effective, but creating serious complications. Fauci, Co-chairman of the council was quoted as saying: "We are adopting a significantly more conservative recommendation profile." One that allows the virus to remain in the body longer in return for sparing the patient from the potential toxicity overload associated with many of the drugs used for treatment. In others words: *If there are no symptoms, don't treat it!* With each year that passes, we are finding out just how effective Nutritional therapy can be, especially when combined with other therapies such as: Stress Management, Healthier Life Style changes and Herbal recommendations.

These combined therapies can play a vital role not only in extending one's life, but also in the quality of life itself!

Note: As of this writing, and after Bernie's doctor telling him to "Die on his own time, if he continued to chose not to take the medications he was prescribing, Bernie got a new Infectious disease physician. This physician is open-minded and looking at Bernie's lab results agrees that Bernie does not require any medication at this time. And furthermore, he felt that the previous doctor's actions and words could have made him liable for a malpractice suit, had there been a witness to his words.

Bernie is to be admired for his courage in sticking to what he believes in. Faith and determination can carry us through the rough times!

****

In Bernie's own words
(2003)

Renders Wellness
1540 Mays Landing Road,
E.H.T., New Jersey 08234

Dear Eileen;

    Since learning and applying your principals and
methods of herbal therapies, my life has improved
tremendously in quality. Eight years ago I did not think
that I could feel as energetic and alive as I do now.

    I thank you for your friendship and sharing your
precious gift with me.

      Sincerely,

      Bernie

FOURTEEN

CANCER

To begin to define what cancer *is* today could fill the pages of many journals. For example, there are as many types of cancer as there are causes. Too, there are of course, the many methods of treatment. A few of the more common forms of cancer are skin, breast, lung and prostate. And there are the cancers that are not as common such as brain cancer, Leukemia and bone cancer. There are cancers that metastasize and spread quickly, and there are cancers that are very slow growing and do not metastasize. For the past forty years billions of dollars have gone into cancer research in hopes of finding a cure. Now in the year 2004 there still remains no promise of a cure in the near future! Though we are finding better and more tolerable treatment methods, our best defense in the fight against cancer is *prevention!*

This may be possible only because of what research findings have uncovered for us to date.
Research studies are now pointing to many common factors that increase our risk of getting cancer in our lifetime. Some of those causes are referred to in a book "The Cancer Dictionary" by Roberta Altman and Michael J. Sarg, M.D. Associate Chief of Medical Oncology, St. Vincent's Hospital, New York City and

Associate Professor of Clinical Medicine, New York
Medical College.

Gathering their information, they inform us in the
Cancer Dictionary of various suspected carcinogens,
which many of us may, or may not be aware of, such
as:

Agent Orange ~ Arsenic ~ Artificial Sweeteners
Asbestos ~ Ascites ~ Aspartame
Azathioprine ~ Benzene ~ Benzidine
Bis (Chlormethl Ether)
Caffeine ~ Chromium
Conjugated Equine Estrogen
CTX ~ Cytoxan
Decaffeinated coffee DES (Diethylstilbestrol)-
Drinking Water (some)
Electromagnetic fields--Endoxan
Environmental tobacco smoke
ETS ~ passive smoke
Fat
Food Additives
Formaldehyde
Hair Dye
Herbicides
Hazardous Waste Sites
Involuntary Smoking
IAQ (indoor air quality)
Melphalan
Methoxsalen
Mouthwash
Microwave oven
Mustard Gas
Nitrate
Nitrite

Nitrosamines
Radon
Nuclear Power Plant
Phenacetin
Saccharin
Smokeless Tobacco
Thorium Dioxide
Vinyl Chloride
Ultraviolet Radiation
2-Naphthylamine

Some of the compounds in the above list may surprise some of us while proving to be confusing to others. However, empowerment begins with understanding (knowledge is power). It opens up the door of opportunity in that it allows us to better manage our health. One way that we can accomplish this is through elimination of, or avoidance of suspected carcinogens.

By no means is the above list of carcinogens considered a complete list. It is in my opinion however, a good start. Yet we have only just begun to recognize potentially harmful compounds, especially when they look great and taste good!

In attempting to treat cancer, the physician must ascertain the type of cancer, the staging and the aggressiveness of treatment he/she believes will successfully combat the cancer, as well as the treatment duration.

What we now know about various drugs often used in chemotherapy for the treatment of cancer is that they are all non-discriminatory in that they do not simply attack and kill cancer cells. They will also attack and kill normal healthy cells. Therefore, the result is that some individuals in cancer therapy may become more vulnerable to anemia, or leukemia. Other common symptoms associated with drug therapy are fatigue, nausea, anorexia and diarrhea can also contribute to a further weakening of the immune system.

However, many Oncologists often fail to recognize how many of these patients are excellent candidates for *Nutritional therapy*. Common sense should tell us that nutritional support with concentrated potencies of specific nutrients might stimulate the production of healthy red blood cells. And those patients (receiving nutritional support) might be better able to proceed through treatment showing increased strength and stamina. While aggressive cancers with bleak prognoses often require aggressive treatment, it should not be dismissed as the fact remains: Potent (strong and often toxic) drugs used to treat aggressive cancers often bring with them a whole new set of health problems that need to be addressed, such as liver toxicity! Again let it be known that nutritional support and herbal medicine has been shown (when recommendations are made by someone with a proven expertise in that field) to assist the body in releasing or removing these toxins from the body!

Understanding then how Nutritional therapy can assist the cancer patient in stimulating the production of healthy new red blood cells, as well as in detoxification could foster a plan that would make Nutritional therapy available for all interested patients! There are many benefits available through Nutritional therapy, and the day will soon come soon when each patient will be allowed just such an option as part of their care.

Armed with this knowledge, why would anyone contemplate going through cancer treatment without the support of other practitioners who can assist in the healing process? Could it be that because bureaucratic policy dictates whether or not, or who will be entitled to take advantage of these services through Insurance policy? Ignorance is not always bliss!

Who better is most qualified to assist these individuals with Nutritional support and Herbal recommendations than a qualified Nutritionist, a Doctor of Naturopathy, or Licensed Naturopath?

While some ND'S are able to be licensed in several states such as Florida, District of Columbia and other states, the laws governing this licensing are not uniform and there are states who do not provide licensing.

Because these practitioners are not licensed, they are often not recognized in all as states as professionals. Therefore, doctors and/or hospitals guide many patients toward their in-house dietitians. Although dietitians do have their place in healthcare, the services rendered by the dietitian, naturopath or nutritionist does not overlap, nor does one undermine the other.

The Doctor of Naturopathy is obliged to have a B.S. prior to enrolling in any College to pursue a degree of Doctor of Naturopathy. Upon completion of studies and earning a degree, it is imperative to obtain sufficient professional Liability Insurance, a license whenever appropriate, and demonstrate an ability to effectively perform their specialty. Each individual must also be provided a disclosure notice of the ND'S specialties and limitations at the time service is rendered.

Why would Insurance Companies not want such practitioners to become part of their Provider Services, especially in realizing that health maintenance/disease prevention could save millions of dollars in money a year previously spent on costly surgeries and chemotherapy, or simply by lowering cancer incidence?

These types of services might offer a more cost effective and safer type of cancer treatment.

Because the Doctor of Naturopathy is not an M.D., they do not (for the most part) fall under the regulation of the American Medical Association. They are not employed by hospitals, nor governed by any Medical Board. In other words, licensing is not obligatory. Therefore they do not write prescriptions, or add to any revenue earned by huge Pharmaceutical Corporations. However, they do often write scripts for nutraceuticals. It is our belief that when managed by a professional, they are non-toxic and non-addictive and most often, proven to be without side effects.

Medical physicians on the other hand, do examine, diagnose and prescribe, and often perform invasive treatments. Therefore, they are obliged by Law to be licensed within the state where they practice. They also are obliged to retain huge amounts of professional liability Insurance. Many individuals now believe that the Pharmaceutical Companies are the richest and most powerful (did I mention influential) Corporations in the world today. They carry a lot of weight and are fully backed by the American Medical Association. In other words, doctors are the practitioners prescribing the drugs manufactured by them and are therefore, supporting these huge conglomerate corporations.

Under normal conditions, the dietitian works under Medical physicians, or in a Hospital setting where they are usually employed. A Dietitian's role is quite different from that of the Doctor of Naturopathy. It is our hope that we have been able to shed some light into these two specialties and show exactly how they work independently of one another.

Dietitians for all intent and purpose are there to control one's diet according to their specific disorder, or disease. For example, special considerations need to be given to the diabetic and/or heart patient. They may manage for instance, the number of calories and fat in the diet of an obese individual who must lose weight in order to save his/her life! They may restrict the Sodium intake for a heart disease patient who has demonstrated a hypersensitivity to Sodium that can increase the blood volume and thus, raise the blood pressure, all of which adds to the patient's risk for heart attack or stroke. Their expertise is of benefit, but different from that of the Doctor of Naturopathy who will strengthen one's constitution through nutritional support, immune enhancement, hormone balancing, detoxification, or recommendations for management of a common disorder for which most of us suffer and for which

105

there are no cures. Disorders such as arthritis, hyperlipidemia (high blood lipid levels), allergies, Chronic Fatigue Syndrome, and other similar disorders.

It is important to make that distinction. And while this type of nutrition is qualified, it will not become part and parcel of our country's Health Coverage Package until we demand it!

More importantly, many of us are unknowingly being deceived, in that we do not understand the distinction between a dietitian and a nutritionist or Dr. of Naturopathy.

This distinction is important because only through recognizing these differences can we realize that we are being discriminated against because our very freedom of choice is not being extended to us! In part, choosing a practitioner of choice is also what brings comfort and confidence into our plan of treatment. Regardless of our choice, M.D., N.D., Dietitian or Nutritionist, the choice should be ours!

An example of how this occurs might be when a patient request nutritional counseling and is provided with referrals only to dietitians.

While the Doctor of Naturopathy is slowing gaining strength in numbers and making their specialty more understood, the transition has been an uphill battle all the way. Yet we are beginning to see the summit.

Although the odds have been stacked against us (Doctors of Naturopathy), it has not prevented hundreds of thousands of individuals from seeking out the aid of Alternative Medicine practitioners year after year. It should also be understood however, that alternative medicine practitioners are not necessarily utilized as "Complimentary" practitioners any longer, at least not in most instances. U.S. in fact is one of the few countries that do not utilize nutrition, or herbs, including several other modalities as their primary medicine. For example, many times when a patient's symptoms cannot be diagnosed, regardless of how much investigative Lab work is done, they are simply sent home. Perhaps that is because many such patients fall into an overlooked category that I refer to as the *gray area.*

This is an area that falls toward the low end of a predetermined scale of what is believed to be acceptable, or disease free! Yet the patient insists all is not well as symptoms continue to persist! However, experience has shown that these persistent symptoms are often a cautionary, or warning stage when symptoms occur just before disease is detectable! It is a fact that we all know of individuals who have complained of nothing more than fatigue long before their cancer was diagnosed. Headaches can often precede an aneurysm, or an oxygen shortage may be the only symptom prior to a heart attack!

Often times, nutritional deficiencies present symptoms before the onset of a disorder. And hormonal imbalances can present symptoms that are also, not readily detectable by the primary care physician. But the specialized Nutritionist can provide

107

help, as this is their field of expertise. We would not want to see a Cardiologist when we are seeking treatment for Arthritis any more than we would see a Gynecologist for treatment of allergies.

While there are medical physicians who may perceive the new nutritional therapy specialist at best as unqualified, perhaps the Dr. of Naturopathy is sometimes also perceived as overstepping his/her boundaries!

We are not however, invading unknown territory, but perhaps only in the minds of the ignorant. Fortunately we pioneers however, are being embraced with open arms and open minds by many of today's new medical graduates. Especially to those who ordinarily do not normally ascribe to drug therapy as the first line of defense. That might include surgeons, chiropractors or osteopaths. The new generation of physicians just coming out of Medical College obviously have been learning new methods of treatment with regard to that gray area of medicine that has for too long been ignored.

For it is in that area, and in that very crucial time of a patient's symptoms wherein disease might be prevented, and when proper intervention might best be applied. If our goal is to better detect the internal problem and make corrections. Not with drugs, but possibly through correction of nutritional deficiencies, restoring hormonal balance, detoxification and immune enhancement. Stress management and exercise are also an import part of each individual's psyche.

Today many of the health books authored by Nutritionists and ND'S can be readily found in Universities and Hospitals around the world. Several of my own titles have often been seen at The Children's Hospital of PA. and in their Library.

Renders Wellness is extremely proud to have been reviewed and accepted through referrals by several Oncologists (Pediatric Div.) at THE CHILDREN'S HOSPITAL OF PA. We worked with several of the children to detoxify, nutritionally support and for immune enhancement.

There is a Research Corporation now dedicated to, if not the prevention of certain types of cancer, (such as breast cancer) certainly in reducing the risk! They are the manufacturers of a product know as Brevail, a naturally-occurring lignan secoisolariciresinol diglucoside (SDG.) See Resource section in back for finding this product.

FIFTEEN

The Immune System

The immune system is comprised of many integral parts that work together. However, for the sake of simplicity we will take a look at the two major parts: Glands, Lymph system and cells.

To begin with, glands contain epithelial cells that are specific for synthesizing compounds that are secreted either into ducts or into the blood. Whenever simple compounds enter a gland's cells via the bloodstream, chemical reactions within the cells build them up into a more complex compound that is incorporated into that particular gland's secretion. For instance: A single cell might constitute a gland. Goblet cells in the mucous lining of the intestines and part of the respiratory tract are known as unicellular glands. The majority of glands however are multicellular, meaning that they are composed of many cells.

Multicellular glands are of two main types: Endocrine (ductless) and exocrine (duct glands). The *Endocrine glands* secrete into the capillaries of the blood, and the *exocrine glands* secrete their compounds into ducts that open up on the surface of the epithelium. The Exocrine glands are of two main types: Simple glands having only one duct, and compound glands when they have more than one duct.

If you are not confused yet, consider this: Simple compound glands are further classified according to the shape of the secretory position of the gland, as either tubular (tube-shaped) or alveolar (sac-shaped).

While the human body contains many glands such as: Thyroid gland, parathyroid glands, adrenal glands, pancreatic glands, ovaries in females and testes in males, pineal gland, thymus, gastric and intestinal mucosa as well as the pituitary that all release their specific hormones, lets take a look at those glands thought to be most involved in the immune response.

Thymus gland ~ This gland is thought to be the primary organ of the lymphatic system. Therefore, as a major component of the body's overall immune system, the endocrine function of the thymus is not only important but also essential. The thymus releases a hormone known as thymosin that is biologically an active peptide that works with other peptides that has a serious responsibility in the maturing and development of the immune system. For example: An individual diagnosed with an impaired thymic function, injections of thymosin will increase the growth of lymphocytes known as "T cells".

T-cells play a major role in activating the immune system's response. In other words it is the thymus that provides an environment in which T-cells mature and learn to distinguish self from oneself during fetal and early postnatal stages. Furthermore, most of the cells that enter into the thymus are destroyed.

T-cell clones that react strongly to self and/or those that do not recognize self are deleted in a process known as negative selection. Other T-cell clones that do recognize self and do not react strongly against self are positively selected.

Whenever these cloned T-cells have passed their test (so to speak) during early training, they soon become part of a larger group of mature T-cells and will eventually reside primarily in peripheral lymph organs for the purpose of recirculating in the blood and lymph.

DiGeorge's Syndrome is a congenital thymic hypoplasia caused by the partial or total absence of cell-mediated immunity resulting from a deficiency of T lymphocytes. It characteristically produces life-threatening hypocalcaemia that may be associated with cardiovascular and facial anomalies. Patients rarely live beyond age 2 without fetal thymic transplant, however prognosis improves when fetal thymic transplant, correction of hypocalcaemia, and repair of cardiac anomalies are possible.

The Spleen ~ This organ is located in the left hypochondrium directly below the diaphragm and just above the left kidney and descending colon, and behind the fundus of the stomach.

After many theories by many experienced physiologists, the spleen is considered to have several functions: Hemopoiesis (the production of blood cells that replaces aged blood cells), defense and serves as a reservoir for blood.

112

While the spleen has many beneficial functions, it is not vital to life. It is invaluable however, in times of stress due to hemorrhage.

Lymph system ~ There is so much that can be written regarding the Lymph system not only because of what it does, but also because of its uniqueness. The lymphatic system is a specialized circulatory system that involves circulating fluid known as lymph that is delivered from the blood and tissue fluid, including a group of vessels (lymphatics) that return the lymph to the blood by a roundabout route. Also included in the lymph system other than the lymph fluid and lymphatic vessels, the lymph system has lymph nodes that are located along the paths of the collecting lymphatic vessels. These lymph nodes or nodules are specialized lymphatic organs and can be found in the intestinal wall (Peyer's patches), and include the tonsils, thymus and spleen.

Lymph is a clear, transparent fluid found in the lymphatic vessels. Interstitial fluid is that fluid which fills spaces in between cells, and it is not the clear transparent fluid it seems to be. For instance, studies have shown that it is a complex and organized constituent. Apparently, it has been shown to have several uses in that it can actually be part of a semi fluid ground substance in some tissues, and in others it is the bound water in a gelatinous ground substance. This interstitial fluid together with blood plasma is exactly what constitutes the extra cellular fluid that

113

comprises the internal environment of the body, that according to one expert, Claude Bernard.

Both lymph and interstitial fluid closely resemble blood plasma in composition. A main difference noted however, is that they have a smaller percentage of proteins than does plasma. Lymph and interstitial fluid is nearly identical when comparisons are made between the two fluids taken from the same area of the body. Further investigation however, found that samples taken from the thoracic duct contains about twice the amount of protein as that taken from most interstitial fluid samples. More than one half of the nearly 3,000 ml of daily lymph flows through the thoracic duct from both the liver and the small intestine.

Lymphatic vessels originate as microscopic blind-end vessels called lymphatic capillaries. Others that originate in the villi of the small intestine are called lacteals.

The wall of the lymphatic capillary consists of a single layer of flattened endothelial cells; very small connective tissue filaments connect capillary cell ends to surrounding cells. This network of lymphatic capillaries are found in the intercellular spaces and largely distributed throughout the body. And although lymphatic and blood capillary networks lie side by side, they are independent of one another. Just as the branches of a single tree independently grow their own leaves, but are not independent of the tree, so too do capillaries work independently, but not without the smooth functioning of the entire system.

The lymph drainage is accomplished in a curious manner as the right upper quadrant of the body allows lymph drainage to occur through various lymph capillaries while the remainder of the body provides for lymph drainage via the thoracic duct. Although these lymph capillaries do resemble veins in structure, their walls are thinner, contain more valves and also contain lymph nodes that are located at various locations along their course. There is also evidence that in the event of damage, most lymph vessels have the capacity for repair or regeneration.

Lymphatic vessels play a vital function in maintaining an internal homeostatic balance. For instance, the high degree of their permeability allows for the admittance of large molecular weight substances of matter, molecules that cannot be absorbed and/or excreted by the blood capillary. The lymphatic system (capillaries) allows the proteins that accumulate in the tissue spaces to be returned to the blood system via the lymph capillaries. This is a vital function to life itself. For if anything hinders the lymphatic return, blood protein concentration and blood osmotic pressure soon fall below normal and fluid imbalance and death will result.

While there is no muscular pumping organ connected with the lymphatic vessels to force lymph (like the heart's pumping action for the blood vessels) the moving action of the lymph fluid, it moves slowly and steadily along its vessels. Lymph flows through the thoracic duct and reenters the general circulation at the rate of 125 ml per hour. And this occurs despite the fact that it flows upward against gravity..

Lymph nodes ~

The Lymph nodes (or glands) are oval in shape and vary in size from that of a pinhead to those that are as large as a lima bean. Lymph moves into the nodes through several afferent lymphatic vessels. These nodes are densely inhabited with lymphocytes, the major component of lymphatic tissue.

Although the majority of lymph nodes occur in groups in specific areas, there are however, a few single nodes.

Locations ~ Submental *and submaxillary groups* are found in the floor of the mouth allowing lymph flow from the nose, lips and teeth.

Superficial cervical glands ~ These nodes are located in the neck along the sternocleidomastoid muscle and allow drainage from the head and neck.

Superficial cubital or supratrochlear nodes ~ Are located just above the bend of the elbow, thus allowing lymph to pass from the forearm.

Axillary nodes ~ Found deep within the armpit and upper chest area forming a cluster of approximately 20 to 30, these nodes are often considerably larger in size as they permit lymph flow to pass from the upper arm, upper part of the thoracic wall, including the breast.

Inguinal nodes ~ Located in the groin area, these nodes allow lymph to flow from the leg and external genitals for drainage.

Functions

Two unrelated functions are carried out by the lymph nodes: Defense and hemopoiesis. Hemopoiesis is the production of blood cells and platelets, a function that is carried out throughout one's lifetime. Hemopoiesis is necessary in order to replace aged cells with new cells.

In their defense mode, lymph nodes provide both filtration and phagocytosis.

Because of the structure of the sinus channels within the lymph nodes, they are able to slow down the flow and it is this action which provides the reticuloendothelial cells that line the channels time to remove microorganisms and other harmful particles. For instance – that would include both cancer cells and/or soot. However a potential problem can occur whenever huge amounts of microorganisms enter into the nodes that the phagocytes cannot fully destroy, thus rendering them unable to prevent further damage. An example of that might be when particles of a malignant tumor breaks away and enters into the lymphatics and travel to the lymph nodes where they may set up new growths.

Cells ~

Earlier on we talked about the Lymph nodes in a previous chapter. In that chapter we mentioned the process known as *Hemopoiesis*, and now we will elaborate a bit further in telling you that there are hemopoietic stem cells that are thought to develop before birth either in the liver or in bone marrow. In infants Immature B cells are developed (probably in the liver) by the time the infant has reached two or three months old. The Second stage of B cell development usually takes place in the lymph nodes and spleen, but only under certain conditions.

B-cells ~ Originally and prior to a B-cell, there are what is known as Immature B-cells which are small lymphocytes containing antibody molecules embedded in their cytoplasmic membranes. Antigens bind to antibodies in these Immature B-cell cytoplasmic membranes and this takes place mainly in lymph nodes and the spleen.

Activated B-cells ~ Once these Immature B-cells become activated they are known as mature, or activated B-cells and they are capable of cloning themselves. They have what is known as memory cells. In other words when an individual is exposed to a set of pathogens to which they have previously been exposed to, these activated B-cells rapidly develop into plasma cells secreting huge amounts of Antibodies which help to create immunity and/or prevent disease.

Formation and types ~ Hemopoietic stem cells are destined to become lymphocytes and follow either one

118

of two developmental pathways, and differentiate into two major classes of lymphocytes--B-lymphocytes and/or T-lymphocytes, or B cells and T cells.

T-Cells ~ by definition, T cells are lymphocytes that have made a detour through the thymus gland before migrating to the lymph nodes and spleen. During their stay in the thymus, stem cells develop into thymocytes, or cells that proliferate as rapidly as any cells found in the body. Thymocytes undergo mitosis three times a day, and as a result their numbers increase enormously in a relatively short time. Mitosis is a type of cell division in which a single cell produces two genetically identical daughter cells. It is the way in which new body cells are produced for both growth and repair.

They stream out of the thymus into the blood and find their way to a new location in other areas of the lymph nodes and spleen called thymus-dependent zones. From this time forward they are then known as T cells.

Similarly to B cells, T cells display antigen receptors on its surface membrane, however these receptors are sites on as yet unidentified molecules-presumably, not immunoglobulins but perhaps compounds similar to them. As for B cell receptors, they differ inasmuch as they are known to be the combining sites of immunoglobulin molecules.

When an antigen encounters a T cell whose surface receptors fit the antigen's epitopes, the antigen selects that T cell by binding to its receptors. This activates or sensitizes the T cell, causing it to initiate a series of reactions. The first reaction is that the sensitized T cell divides repeatedly to form a clone of identical sensitized T cells. All of these sensitized T cells then release chemical compounds into the surrounding tissues that are collectively known as *lymphokines*. Lymphokines are of individual types such as: Chemo tactic factor, migration inhibition factor, macrophage activating factor and lymphotoxin.

All of these lymphokines have distinctive responsibilities with regard to their integral part of the body's defense line. A brief overview is as follows:

Chemo tactic factor ~ These lymphokines attract macrophages, leading hundreds of them to converge into the vicinity of the antigen-bound sensitized T cell.

Migration inhibition factor ~ These lymphokines literally stops the migration of macrophages. *Macrophage activating factor* ~ At this point, lymphokines work by prodding any assembled macrophages in order to destroy their antigens by phagocytosing them at a rapid rate.

Lymphotoxin ~ This is a potent poison able to quickly kill any cell that it attacks. Hence, this is the lethal substance that has earned sensitized T-cells the nickname of "killer cells."

Distribution sites

Obviously, huge populations of lymphocytes can be found in the structures where they are formed and multiply, namely in the bone marrow, thymus gland, lymph nodes and spleen.

Note: Much more can be said regarding the chemistry or biochemistry of man, and if interested one might include the textbook reading of "Anatomy and physiology" by Anthony and Thibodeau, with several editions by The C.V. Mosby Co.

Recommendations for the Immune system

Vitamin A ~ This vitamin aids in the growth and repair of body tissues and helps maintain smooth, soft, disease-free skin. Internally it helps to protect the mucous membranes of the mouth, nose, throat, and lungs, thereby reducing susceptibility to infection. A fat-soluble vitamin that can be toxic when taken in excess, I prefer and always recommend its partner Beta-carotene, as this supplement is non-toxic as

it is released into the body as needed in a time-release manner. 25,000 I.U's is recommended daily.

Selenium ~ This is an essential mineral that is known to kill free radicals due to its antioxidant powers, and help to reduce the risk of cancer. However, more in not better, and Selenium toxicity is possible causing many symptoms, including severe hair loss. It also works with vitamin E to promote normal body growth and fertility. It is necessary for the production of prostaglandin, a substance that can affect blood pressure. 350 micrograms daily is recommended for adults, and not to exceed 700 micrograms. Organic Selenium (dimethyl selenium) is non-toxic and the preferred form.

Zinc ~ Zinc is another mineral that works as an antioxidant and is also necessary for prevention, or reducing the risk of certain types of cancer. Laboratory studies using animals have shown that the vitamins A, C, E, and B1, the minerals Selenium and Zinc have prevented development of cancers. They are able to do this by stimulating the body's immune system. Free radicals (cancer causing agents) are chemicals produced by the body when exposed to harmful substances such as radiation, food and drink contamination, rancid fats, and air pollution.

Zinc, vitamin C, and the herb Bilberry when taken consistently can prevent or delay cataracts.

Recommendations: The turnover of body zinc has been calculated from radioisotope studies to be 6 milligrams per day, an amount that needs to be replaced. The

RDA for zinc is 15 milligrams, which takes into consideration that only about 40 percent (6 milligrams) will be absorbed from food by the body.

CHAPTER SIXTEEN
Recipes and Suggestions
Beverages (healthy)

Water ~ It is advisable that every household have a Water Test completed in order to determine its mineral content, as well as present organisms.

Homeowners can pick up a guide showing tolerable Minerals and organisms from their local Health Department, or at the Department of Environmental Protection Agency in order to make the comparison Of what is an "Allowable percentage" for their Specific area, and what is actually present in one's Drinking water.

Your Yellow Page Directory of telephone numbers will provide that listing. There are other Laboratories in most areas, that will provide independent Testing is for a nominal fee of about $10.00, or there about.

Seltzer water is an alternative

Vitamin water (see Resource section)

Green Chinese Oolong green tea with pure water. Studies confirm original findings that this tea contains polyphenols, one in particular, catechins has been shown to stimulate the production of white T-cells, thus providing immune enhancement ability.

Concentrated (unsweetened) fruit juices ~ double diluted with water is good.

Protein drinks ~ These include Soy and whey. They are excellent when combined with fruit, such as in a blender or Smoothie machine.

Almond milk ~ Soymilk ~ Rice milk ~ Goat's milk

Homemade Lemonade or iced tea
    Avoid high content sugar drinks, such as sodas. Excess sugar intake inhibits the body's ability to store and keep available many essential nutrients, including the essential B+ Complex vitamins.

Note: Cow's milk is high in fat and also contains synthetic hormones that the Barnyard animals have been fed.

Recipes
Beans and Rice

Ingredients

1 tablespoon of Extra virgin olive oil

1 small green pepper

1 celery stalk

1 small onion

1 clove of fresh garlic

1 cup of pre-cooked rice

*Preferably a combination of wild and white, or brown

1 large fresh tomato diced

1 can of red kidney beans (8 to 10 oz. Can)

½ cup of Sherry cooking wine

- Optional – 1 cup of diced "lite" Polish kielbasa

Directions

In a large skillet dice and add first five ingredients one at a time.

Cook on low h eat for about 5 minutes

Add kielbasa and simmer for a few more minutes

Add diced tomato and stir

Rinse and combine kidney beans and blend

Add water as needed

Simmer on low heat for an additional five minutes

Finally, add cooking wine before serving

Serve with salad

Note: Either beans and rice or corn and rice makes a complete perfect protein meal.

Bread sticks (Yucca root flour)

This recipe uses gluten free flour that is acceptable for those on Gluten-free diets, and is low in carbohydrates making it good for diabetics! In Brazil, its main ingredients come from the tropical manioc plant, a.k.a. cassava or yucca.

Yucca root flour can be obtained by logging onto Internet and going to www.Chebe.com or by using their Toll free # 1-800-217-9510Fact: While this fact is little known, it is true that rats turn their backs on an opportunity to feast on white flour!

Ingredients

1 pack of Chebe flour (Sold in a Six-pack)

2 tablespoons of extra virgin olive oil

2 large eggs (or eggbeater equivalent)

3 Tablespoons of water

Directions

In a large Mixing bowl slowly combine flour, oil and eggs.

Next: slowly add the water until smooth and blended. Roll flour into sticks about ¾" thick. Place on a non-greased pan.

Bake in a preheated 375-degree oven for approximately 25 minutes. Serve warm.

Suggestions: For your own taste, add onion, jalapeno, cheese or whatever! Or simply sprinkle with garlic before baking.

Breakfast (Ham n eggs)

Ingredients

1 thin slice of Canadian bacon

2 eggs, egg whites or egg beaters

1 slice of Swiss cheese

*Vegetable leftovers

1 tablespoonful of Extra virgin olive oil

Directions

In a skillet add olive oil and any leftover vegetable (boiled potato, peas, broccoli & etc.) and simmer.
Or add green pepper and onion or mushrooms
In another small pan add a teaspoon of olive oil and heat Canadian bacon. When vegetables are warm add two beaten eggs, egg whites or eggbeaters to skillet. Do not stir, and keep on low flame.
Gently lay the slice of Swiss cheese on top of mixture.

Continue to watch and gradually lift perimeter away from pan to prevent sticking. When underside reaches desired color, flip to other side and continue to cook for another minute or so.

Serve with a piece of fruit

Butter (Instead of)

Almond putter

Peanuts and peanut butter contain the highest number of pesticide residues of most other foods found in the Super Market (over 100)

Ghee: cooking butter at medium high heat until completely melted makes this ancient butter. When butter begins to cool again, the fat is skimmed off the top. This provides the flavor without all the fat!

Olive spread ~ Another way to utilize butter is to warm butter in a small pot and after it has melted and is allowed to sit and cool, combine equal amount of Extra virgin olive oil and blend. Allow to set.

Some recipes, including whipped potatoes, cookies pies and etc. will work well by adding low fat cream cheese, or low fat Sour cream for replacing some of the butter.

Tahini can be substituted in some recipes for peanut butter.

Cheesecake can become healthy and tasty by using silken tofu, lemon and low-fat cream cheese together with low fat Ricotta cheese!

Let your imagination open the door to new and healthier recipes!

Corn bread

Ingredients

1 cup of corn meal

½ cup of cornstarch

½ cup of potato or tapioca starch flour

½ cup of gluten free flour

½ teaspoon of Sea salt

2 Teaspoons of Aluminum-free (Featherweight brand) baking powder that can be found at your local Health Food Store

2- Tablespoons of Extra virgin oil

2 whole eggs beaten

1 cup of canned goat milk

½ cup of butter

- Optional ¼ cup of cook corn, ¼ cup of walnuts,
- Jalapeno pepper

Directions

In a large mixing bowl add first six ingredients (dry ingredients) and blend well.

Add eggs, butter and oil and continue to blend

Add milk and any other optional ingredients and continue to stir until well blended.

Bake in a preheated oven at 375 degrees for 25 minutes, or until lightly brown on top

Serve warm or pan fry the next day!

French fries

Ingredients

2 to 3 large Russet Idaho potatoes

1 Tablespoonful of extra virgin olive oil

Spike seasoning

Directions

Wash, peal and slice the potatoes lengthwise about ½" wide for each slice

Spread out on a cookie sheet lined with baking paper.

Using a Baker's brush, lightly brush each French fry with the oil.

Sprinkle with your favorite Spike Seasoning

Bake at 375-degree oven for about 20 to 25 minutes

Suggestion: When time is of the essence, microwave the potatoes for five minutes before peeling and this will cut down on the amount of baking time required.

This eliminates the chemicals and high Sodium often found in prepared French fries!

Suggestion :If time is of the essence, microwave the potatoes for 5 minutes before pealing and this will cut down on the amount of baking time required.

This eliminates chemicals and high Sodium found in prepared French fries!

Lunch suggestions

~ Homemade soups

~ Yogurt and a piece of fruit

~ Eggbeater or Egg white omelet

~ Salad with protein (chicken, tuna, egg)

~ Vegetable platter

~ Fruit and a small Salad

~ Protein drink with fruit

Oils

~ Extra virgin olive oil

~ Almond oil (great for doing pie crusts)

~ Sesame oil

~ Safflower oil

~ Ghee

~ Sautee with low sodium chicken bouillon

Pie Crust

Ingredients

1 cup of garbanzo bean flour (Specialty Stores or on the Internet.) Or substitute 1 cup of Gluten free flour

1 cup of Brown rice flour or Almond meal

1 cup of Almond oil

White flour has little or no nutritional value and can
trigger allergic response in many people. It is also
The only food avoided by rats!

Raw almonds or Almond meal is highly nutritious and low in carbohydrates with only 1 gram of saturated fat to an ounce. Next to Olive oil, Almond oil is highest in monounsaturated fats that are said to lower LDL cholesterol without lowering the "good" HDL levels. Almond oil may be less popular than some oils because it is higher in price and requires refrigeration. Almonds are high in potassium. Magnesium, phosphorus and protein. Cancer clinics often recommend patients take 10 to 12 raw almonds per day because of their laetrile content. Laetrile acts as an anti-cancer agent. Both almond oil and almond butter are nutritious.

Directions

Mix flours and oil together in a Mixing bowl
Knead with hands until it forms a ball
Break into two pieces and with your hands press into pie pan.

Using your favorite filling, follow directions and bake in a preheated oven at 375 degrees for about 25 to 25 minutes.

Pizza Crust

Ingredients
1 packet of Chebe yucca flour
1 egg
water ¼ cup
Oil ~ 1-Tablespoon

Directions

Flour surface of your cooking counter as well as your rolling pin. Roll dough out on top of cooking paper. When it is large enough lay pie pan on top of rolled . dough and using the cooking paper, flip over. Trim sides and ripple with thumb. Bake for 15 to 20 minutes until lightly browned in a preheated 375-degree oven. Remove promptly and add favorite toppings.
Return to warm oven and continue to cook for another 10 minutes or so, or until toppings are begin to bubble.

Potato (healthier replacements for)

Broccoli and cheese

Fried cabbage and onions

Spaghetti squash

Wild rice

Cauliflower and cheese

Sweet potato

Brown rice

Corn and rice or beans and rice

Mashed medley (1 large potato, 2 carrots, 1 apple and 1 turnip)

Protein choices

Eggs

Cheese (goat cheese, low fat Ricotta)

Yogurt

Beans and rice

Corn and rice

Chicken

Protein shakes

Fish

Lean, top choice cut of red meat with fat trimmed

Pork

Garbanzo beans (rinsed and placed in a shallow baking pan. Add I tablespoon of Extra virgin olive oil and your favorite herb (Cayenne). Bake in a pre-heated 375-degree oven for approximately 20 minutes, or until beans begin to turn golden brown. 9 grams of protein per ½ cup serving!

Shrimp Casserole

Ingredients

¾ pound of large fresh shrimp

1 cup of Uncle Ben's or Basmati rice (precooked)

1 Tablespoon of Extra Virgin Olive oil

2 stalks of celery

1 small onion

1 small pepper (red, green or yellow)

1 tsp. of roasted garlic

½ to 1 Teaspoon of Turmeric

½ Teaspoon of Curry

2 Medium sized ripe tomatoes (chopped)

Leftover vegetables, or vegetable of your choice: Squash, corn, and peas!

Grated Parmesan

Directions

In a large skillet, add Olive oil, chopped celery, onion, pepper and garlic and cook slowly for about 5 minutes, or until onion turns translucent.

Add unpeeled fresh shrimp and continue to cook slowly. Mix in chopped tomatoes, Turmeric and Curry and continue to cook on low heat, stirring occasionally. Begin to add in rice and keep mixture moist by adding water as needed, or white cooking wine.
The last step is to add in precooked vegetables of choice
Sprinkle with Parmesan cheese before serving!

Soup Base
2 quarts of water
Low Sodium chicken or beef bullion
Directions
Add two quarts of water to a large pot
Mix Soup bullion and then add to pot

Starter

In a large skillet add one tablespoonful of Olive oil

1 mall onion chopped

1 stalk of celery

Green pepper (optional)

½ teaspoonful of roasted crushed garlic (can be purchased at your Supermarket)

When vegetables become translucent, add into bullion mix that has been simmering in a large pot.

To complete your favorite soup

When soup has been cooking on low heat for about 15 minutes, add in rice, potato, carrot, chicken, beef, or any of your favorite meats and/or vegetables.

Continue cooking for another twenty minutes. Turn burner off and allow soup to cool gradually. Reheat when ready to eat!

Sugar replacements

~ Frozen concentrated white grape juice concentrate
(Look for frozen can that is made with 100% juice
Concentrate, and without added sugars.)

~ Date sugar (expensive, use sparingly!) Easily
metabolized by the body, without causing huge
fluctuations in blood sugar levels.

~ Strained baby foods: Applesauce, prunes,
peaches,
Pears. Ideal for baking recipes.

~ ½ cup of raisins steeped in water (just covering
raisins)
Steep raisins in water for about twenty minutes,
and the water will absorb the raisin's sweetness.

~ Stevia (herb)

~ Fresh fruit whenever possible (Replace Pancake
Syrup)
Cook one apple, or banana in ½ cup of Orange
juice

   In a small pan and as it begins to bubble, slowly
add Cinnamon and vanilla to taste and as it cools it will
begin to thicken.

~ Raw or unprocessed honey from the Beehive

~Unsulphured molasses (High in B+ complex vitamins, and other essential minerals).

Vegetable Stew

Ingredients

1-Tablespoonful of Extra Virgin Olive oil

1 Small onion

1 celery stalk

1 small green pepper

1 clove of garlic or 1 teaspoonful of prepared chopped Garlic

1 whole tomato chopped

2 cups of cabbage chopped and par-boiled

1 whole carrot

½ cup of small white beans (Fava)

½ cup of cooked rice

½ cup of low sodium chicken bullion or water

**Optional 2 slices (size of palm) Canadian bacon diced

One (1) teaspoon of Worcestershire sauce

¼ cup of cooking wine

Parmesan cheese

Directions

Add first 5 ingredients to family sized fry pan and simmer for about 5 minutes.

Combine next 5 ingredients slowly, one at a time and continue to cook on a low flame.

Add ½ cup of water or bullion and continue to stir occasionally.

After about 10 minutes of simmering, add Worcestershire sauce

**Optional – final ingredient is cooking wine

Sprinkle dish with grated Parmesan cheese before serving!

Resources

1. Herbal products ~

It is highly recommended that in purchasing any Herbal products discussed in this book should be purchased in its Herbal products are often thought to be safer when purchased from Manufacturers with Laboratories here in the U.S. in order to insure both potency and purity of the specific herb.

Doses: Unless a qualified and credentialed Herbalist or Naturopath is seeing one, follow recommended doses found on container. And *always* Inform your primary care physician of your intent to use any herbal product. Herbs contain essential oils, minerals, phenols, tannin and other compounds that may/or may not be contraindicated in one's particular therapy

2. Vitamins

See your Nutritionist, or Naturopath of Primary Care physician in order to insure that you are taking the proper amount of any essential mineral, in order that you will benefit from supplementing with these essential nutrients. More is not always better, as many might believe. As this kind of inexperienced supplementing can contribute to imbalances of other essential nutrients.

3. Supplements

Your local Health Food Store will be a good source

for purchasing all of your nutritional needs as they most often carry supplements that are without feed dyes and other synthetic compounds.

4. BARLEAN'S at 1-800-445-3529
   Organic Flax Oil ~ High in lignin's (many benefits)
   Also handles various other products, including the
   New Brevail. Brevail is a newly developed breast
   Cancer prevention product (believed to lower risk
   of) and sold through Barlean's. Learn more at
   www.brevail.com

5. Beet root (Betaine) for muscle weakness. The Herb
   House in Banning, CA. Call toll free 1-800-569
   -0686 or (909)-849- 4672.

6. Vitamin Water ~ Energy Brands, Inc. Whitestone,
   N.Y. 1-800-746-0087 to find a Distributor

7. Yucca root flour (packaged for rolls, pizza & etc.)
   www.Chebe.com or call toll free 1-800-217-9510

Bibliography

1. Anatomy and Physiology by Anthony and
   Thibodeau with several editions by C.V. Mosby Co.

2. The Cancer Dictionary copyright 1992
   Facts On File, Inc., New York
   By: Roberta Altman and Michael J. Sarg M.D.
   ISBN: 0-8160-2608-4

3. THE HIV DRUG BOOK Copyright 1995
   Simon Schuster, Inc. ISBN 0-671-53518-8
   Project In form's Guide To The Management of
   Opportunistic Infections by Michael Wright,
   principal author

4. The Holistic Cookbook ISBN: 0-9711551-0-0
   Copyright 2001 Renders Wellness/Publishing
   Eileen Renders N.D. author

5. Methyl Magic by Craig Cooney, Ph.D. (Andrews
   McMeel 1999) Quote "Without methylation there
   would be no life at all."

Index

Accumulative Effect, 12,76, 83
ACMC, 7, 43, 80
ADHD, 1X,50, 54,57
Aluminum, 49,57,62
Am. Cancer Society, 61
Anemia, 52, 65, 89,102
Antagonists, 45,48,60, 64, 75
Antibiotic, 1V, 58,85
Antioxidant, 121,122
Anxiety, 67
Astragalus root, 53,86
AZT, 1, 30, 41-42, 67-69
B+Complex, V111, 49, 63, 124
Bastyr University, 5, 6
Beta Carotene, 121
Betaine, 54
Betaine Hydrochloride, 52
Bernie's Decision, 82,95
Bilberry, 52-53
Biochemistry Profile, 43
Bioflavonoid, 92
Bloating/Gas, 52
Brevail, 109
CD 3'S, 88,92-93
CD 4'S, 89,92,94-94
Calcium/Magnesium, 90
Cancer, 74, 99, 102, 104
Cancer Staging, 101
Candida Albicans, 1V,V, 29 57, 63
Carcinogens, 45,61,101
Cells, 102, 111, 117, 119
Chemotherapy, 101
Chiropractic, 1,5
Cholesterol, 52, 78,96
Chlorophyll, 53
CO-Enzyme-Q-10, 53,90
Colds & Flu, 52
Constipation, 52
Contraindications, 13,44,52
Counseling, 3, 28, 33,44

Dept. of Health & Human Services, 77
Diarrhea, 53, 67, 81
Digestion and- Metabolism, 39, 52
Denatured And Devitalized Foods, 49, 56, 64 65
Detoxification, 44
Dietitians, 103,105
Disease, 17,34
Drug Free, 95
Essential Fatty Acids, 53,59
Energy, 53
Exercise, V1,109
Extra Virgin Olive Oil, 64,130
FDA ~ Food And Drug Administration, 58
Fatigue, 71
Federal Health Panel, 96
Flax Oil, 50-53
Food Additives, 50
Folic Acid, 52,90
Garlic, 86,92
Gen Recommendations, 10,45
Genotyping, 90
Glands, 56, 110,116
Glands, Swollen 84
Guided Imagery, 23,80-82
HIV/AIDS, 1,3,9, 12,16,18,21 27,37,69,77,96
HIV Consortium, 2,7,9,43,80
HIV DRUGS, 67
DDC~ or DIDEOXYCYTIDINE, 68
DDL DIDANOSINE, 69
D4T STAVODINE, 70
FAMCICLOVIR, 71
FOSCARNET, 71
GANCICLOVIR, 72
DRONABINOL, 73
LAMIVUDINE, 72
GROWTH HORMONE, 74
RHGH, 74

MEGESTROL, 75
HIV replication, 2,90,93
Headaches, 42,51,71,81,108
Healthier Food Choices, 49
Heart Disease, 59,96
Herbal Medicine, X1,1,80
Hydrogenated Oils, 50,57,62
Hypersensitivity, 71
Hypertension, V1,42,56,67
89,105
Immune System, 24,35,46,53
56,77-78,102,110
Recommendations for, 122
Infectious Disease Ctr., 10,14
15,84,87,94
Inner Conflict, V111
Inorganic, V11
Insomnia, 42,67,81,88
Intolerable Symptoms, 41
Iodine, X,56
Kidney Disorders, 67,69,71
L-Acidophilus, V
Leukemia, 102
Liver, 1V,15,37,49,54,67,70
76,83
Lymph System, 113,116
Marijuana, 83
Milk thistle, 54
Muscle Weakness, 54,67,81
N.I.H. National Institutes
Of Health, 5,61
National Cancer Inst., 46,57
Natural Healing, 3,35,94
Naturopathy, 7,12,22,106
&107
Nausea, 54,71,88
Nitrosamines, 61-62
Nutrition, 05
Nutrition Deficiencies, 45
108
Nutritional Program, 42,80
Nutritional Therapy, 42,80
97,102
Oxalic Acid, 1X
Peace, Hope &Charity   11

18,21,24,30-31
Phosphoric Acid, 57
Pre-Cancerous Conditions, 47-
48
Progression, Disease, 10,37, 39
48,71,84
Protein, 66
Recipes, 125
Relaxation, 23,39
Probiotic, V
SAMe or
Sadenosylmethionine, 54
Sexually Transmitted Disease,
17, 34
Sodium Chloride, 56, 62
Sore Throat, 54
Steroids, 111
Stress, 05,23,97
Synthetic Hormones, 50-51
124
T-4 Cells, 86
T-Cells, 111
T-Counts, 84
The American Cancer Society,
61
The Cancer Dictionary, 99
The Children's Hospital, 109
Toxins, 111, 11, 28, 37
Trace Minerals, 51
Upper Respiratory Prob., 29,39
Web Site, 59
Weight loss, 105